Ebola's Message

Basic Bioethics
Arthur Caplan, editor

A complete list of the books in the Basic Bioethics series appears at the back of this book.

Ebola's Message

Public Health and Medicine in the Twenty-First Century

edited by Nicholas G. Evans, Tara C. Smith, and Maimuna S. Majumder

The MIT Press
Cambridge, Massachusetts
London, England

This book was set in Stone Sans and Stone Serif by Toppan Best-set Premedia Limited. Printed and bound in the United States of America.

Library of Congress Cataloging-in-Publication Data

Names: Evans, Nicholas G., 1985– , editor. | Smith, Tara C., 1976– , editor. | Majumder, Maimuna S., editor.
Title: Ebola's message : public health and medicine in the twenty-first century / edited by Nicholas G. Evans, Tara C. Smith, and Maimuna S. Majumder.
Other titles: Basic bioethics.
Description: Cambridge, MA : The MIT Press, [2016] | Series: Basic bioethics | Includes bibliographical references and index.
Identifiers: LCCN 2016015018 | ISBN 9780262035071 (hardcover : alk. paper)
Subjects: | MESH: Hemorrhagic Fever, Ebola—prevention & control | Hemorrhagic Fever, Ebola—epidemiology | Communicable Disease Control | Disease Outbreaks | Public Health | Ebolavirus
Classification: LCC RC140.5 | NLM WC 534 | DDC 614.5/7—dc23 LC record available at https://lccn.loc.gov/2016015018

10 9 8 7 6 5 4 3 2 1

Contents

Series Foreword

Glenn McGee and I developed the Basic Bioethics series and collaborated as series coeditors from 1998 to 2008. In Fall 2008 and Spring 2009 the series was reconstituted, with a new Editorial Board, under my sole editorship. I am pleased to present the forty-fifth book in the series.

The Basic Bioethics series makes innovative works in bioethics available to a broad audience and introduces seminal scholarly manuscripts, state-of-the-art reference works, and textbooks. Topics engaged include the philosophy of medicine, advancing genetics and biotechnology, end-of-life care, health and social policy, and the empirical study of biomedical life. Interdisciplinary work is encouraged.

Arthur Caplan

Ebola's Message: A Multidisciplinary Call to Action

Nicholas G. Evans, Tara C. Smith, and Maimuna S. Majumder

It would not be an exaggeration to call the Ebola virus disease (EVD) outbreak an unmitigated disaster, resulting in 28,575 infections and 11,313 deaths as of October 28, 2015.[1] The three countries that bore the overwhelming burden of the disease—Guinea, Liberia, and Sierra Leone—have been devastated. The situation has been complicated by a slow international response; existing vulnerabilities in the health systems of the affected countries as a result of colonialism, civil war, and systemic poverty; and disease emergence in a previously unaffected region of the African continent.

The disaster is, in many ways, one of the developed world's making. The response of the World Health Organization (WHO), charged with global infectious disease mobilization and response, was considered a failure, receiving heavy criticism from groups such as Médicins Sans Frontières, which engaged in outbreak response months before the WHO. The United States government allocated an unprecedented US $6.2 billion for funds to combat the outbreak domestically and internationally; the response, however, has been critiqued for building Ebola treatment centers that were neither staffed nor received patients, operating dangerous clinical trials in affected countries, and reacting to unfounded public panic in a manner that threatened the response effort at large.

Despite the failure to respond appropriately or quickly, there have been promising developments that may improve future responses to infectious disease epidemics, including those caused by Ebola virus. During this outbreak, the world witnessed the Director-General of the WHO brief the UN Security Council for the first time in history, leading to a UN Security Council directive issued about the EVD outbreak—the first time the Security Council has officially commented on a public health event. Fifteen years of biodefense spending by developed nations came to fruition, with the emergence of a series of prospective therapeutic treatments and vaccines for EVD, some of which have returned promising results in clinical trials. And—though perhaps too little, too late—it has been demonstrated that without strong *global* public health systems, epidemics in one part of the world can easily cross national borders.

The 2013–2016 EVD outbreak is perhaps the most significant public health event since the 2003 severe acute respiratory syndrome epidemic and the 2009 H1N1 influenza pandemic; as a result, there now exists a considerable demand for the examination of "lessons learned" from the EVD outbreak and how such lessons might be applied to future infectious disease outbreaks. This volume responds to this demand, but in doing so seeks to inform a broader and—to us—worthwhile project in addressing the problem that arises when a range of otherwise disparate disciplines and fields of inquiry bear on the same problem. In bringing together a *multidisciplinary* set of scholars, this volume illuminates the ongoing EVD outbreak from a range of perspectives in the life sciences, clinical medicine, the social sciences, law, communications, and the humanities.

The Need for Multidisciplinary Links

A central issue in identifying and responding to infectious disease outbreaks is the complex interplay with human societies and infectious diseases. Few would deny that culture plays an important role in health and health care, but it can often be assumed that culture is more or less constant in geographically localized disease outbreaks involving diseases that are a routine part of the health landscape of a given community. Caregivers and policymakers working in their own societies, during the normal periods of illness (including seasonal illnesses, such as influenza), will rarely have to explicitly reflect on their cultural assumptions.

These assumptions fall apart, however, in cases of severe, widespread disease outbreaks. When outbreaks threaten whole societies, as in the case of the H1N1 1918 "Spanish Influenza" outbreak—which infected an estimated one-third of the world's population[2]—or when diseases cross national borders or move between cultural groups, as we have seen with the spread of Middle East respiratory syndrome coronavirus from the Kingdom of Saudi Arabia to South Korea, the background cultural, social, and ethical assumptions behind public health and medicine can break down. The response to EVD faced both of these problems: an outbreak that overwhelmed the countries experiencing the worst of the disease, coupled with international transmission and a global response effort.

This is not the first time in the history of EVD that the tension between society, science, and clinical medicine has presented itself. Barry and Bonnie Hewlett, medical anthropologists invited by the WHO to assist in the 2000 EVD outbreak in Uganda, described the conditions under which the response effort could be self-defeating. The Hewletts found that the disruption of the practice of local burial and funeral customs, distrust of international response teams—even the lack of visibility of patients in treatment centers from the outside—encouraged recidivism and extended the duration of the outbreak.[3]

Fifteen years later, the situation has grown more complex. The 2013–2016 outbreak, to begin, appeared in a novel location on the African continent. Liberia, Guinea, and Sierra Leone had never been the site of an EVD outbreak before, raising questions about the emergence of the virus: Why had the virus appeared here, and *now*? Had Ebola virus emerged in a novel location due to ecological disruption in Western Africa? Had the suspected bat hosts changed their range? Was this a new, more transmissible variant of the virus? Or had it always been present in this region, as hinted at by a 1982 paper in the *Annales de l'Institut Pasteur*?[4] News and social media disseminated huge quantities of misinformation regarding the clinical features of EVD, its potential for spread to other locations, and interventions—from quarantine to essential oils and homeopathy—that could curb the epidemic. Nation states, responding to the possibility of a person infected with Ebola virus crossing their borders, enforced travel restrictions and even denied health care workers travel to affected regions. The return of health care workers infected with Ebola virus to developed nations and the first documented incidence of Ebola virus transmission within the United States fueled fears of a worldwide pandemic. The perceived mismanagement of local cases led the public in the United States to lose trust in local, state, national, and global authorities and their ability to manage the public health response to EVD. This loss of trust lead to the creation of an "Ebola czar" position in the US government. The scientific and medical establishment, bringing with them a range of novel potential treatments for EVD, was quickly mired in controversy attempting to balance the ethics and efficacy of testing new interventions.

As scholars whose work on infectious disease covered one or more dimensions of the 2013–2016 outbreak—and, moreover, scholars actively engaged in public outreach—we experienced much of this debate. There were, no doubt, many causes for the controversies that occurred over 2014 and into 2016, but a clear instigator was a lack of rapport between practitioners and researchers who had a role to play in understanding and responding to the outbreak. Sometimes, clinicians demonstrated little consideration for the social and cultural factors of the individual countries (and in some cases, municipalities) that were most impacted by the EVD outbreak in West Africa. Life scientists and epidemiologists often spoke of the concept of "clinical equipoise"—in which there is no agreement in the expert community about whether one treatment option is better than another—as if it were an uncontroversial guiding light in how to justify and design clinical trials, when the literature on that subject is far from settled. In other instances, government officials, politicians, bioethicists, journalists, and social scientists recommended certain kinds of responses, such as travel restrictions, with little knowledge about the basic scientific properties of the Ebola virus. In all these cases, what was missing was an understanding of something beyond the relatively strict boundaries of a particular field of inquiry.

This book is a response to the problem of a lack of links between disciplines. This is not a *substitute* for diverse interactions and collaborations between researchers, but it is our hope that the following chapters will serve as a way for readers to break the boundaries of their respective wheelhouses and make a start at understanding—and, more importantly, *valuing*—the work of others. Here, Ebola's message is a reminder that responding to a complex infectious disease outbreak requires scientific and clinical knowledge, political acumen, anthropological understanding, bioethical reasoning, and journalistic integrity. No one person can have all of these qualities or learn all of these skills. We need each other.

With this in mind, our selection process for chapters reflects the diversity of the outbreak. Our contributors are bench scientists, physicians, political scientists, public relations experts, lawyers, philosophers, anthropologists, epidemiologists, and communications scholars. They come from a wide variety of professional backgrounds, including government, academia, nongovernmental organizations, and freelance. They are, themselves, in a variety of career stages from students to heads of departments, to high-level government employees, to award-winning journalists. They hail from four continents.

The interdisciplinary nature of this volume, moreover, means that some hard choices had to be made about what ground to cover and what to elide. There is, for example, no chapter on the scientific background to developing the novel therapeutic interventions that have been tested and used during the outbreak. Although our chapters in parts III and V do comment on some of the sociological features of infectious disease outbreaks, we do not have a specific chapter devoted to sociology. And while many of our contributors take time to relate their work or expertise to the functions (and dysfunctions) of the WHO, there is no single chapter devoted entirely to the role of the WHO, the World Health Assembly, and the United Nations Security Council.

Structure of the Volume

This volume is divided into five sections. Part I focuses on the Ebola virus and the management of EVD. In chapter 1, Stephen Goldstein explains the virology of Ebola virus as a member of the *filoviridae* family of viruses. Having established how Ebola infects cells, we move to the clinical management of EVD in resource-rich and resource-poor settings. Patricia Henwood, a two-time veteran of the response effort in Liberia, discusses the challenge of treating EVD in a resource-poor setting in chapter 2, including the unique challenges that EVD presents to caregivers. Michael Connor, Jr. discusses the very recent problem of treating EVD in developed nations in chapter 3, considering the case where resources are plentiful but a lack of knowledge about the disease creates uncertainty about what treatments and supportive care actually work to save patients. Part I enables the reader to distinguish between Ebola as a virus, the disease that virus causes, and the context that makes treating Ebola so challenging.

In part II, the focus moves to delve further into the epidemiology of the outbreak. In chapter 4, Christian Althaus explores the strengths and weaknesses of various mathematical modeling efforts that took place during the epidemic. Then, Daniel Bausch and Lara Schwarz describe how ecology and economics determine the appearance and spread of EVD in chapter 5. Armand Sprecher of Médecins Sans Frontières closes the section in chapter 6 by lending insight into the efforts his organization has made over the past year, how it experienced the spread of Ebola, and the difficulties and frustrations inherent in such work.

In part III, the social, political, and legal contexts of the current outbreak are discussed. In chapter 7, Adia Benton offers insight into the origin stories of Ebola—widely discussed, but often misunderstood—and compares a troubling set of stories that simultaneously assign blame for the epidemic to West Africans while ignoring their violent history at the hands of colonial powers. The legacy of misery and suffering in West Africa is mirrored in Kim Yi Dionne and Laura Seay's account of the history of racist perceptions of West Africa in chapter 8, beginning with an examination of a 2014 *Newsweek* cover blaming the EVD outbreak on the consumption of bushmeat. In chapter 9, Alexandra Phelan examines the legal structure that surrounds infectious disease response and how this fared and failed in the context of an unprecedented epidemic of EVD.

Part IV examines the mainstream and social media response to the outbreak. In chapter 10, Cyril Ibe examines the social media response to the EVD outbreak, as well as the use of social media as a tool during infectious disease epidemics more broadly. In chapter 11, Cristine Russell, drawing on a career writing on infectious diseases from HIV/AIDS in the 1980s through to present day Ebola, presents a journalist's perspective on risk communication in an age of multiple, competing media sources. Marjorie Kruvand completes this part with an examination of the public relations aspect of an epidemic, focusing on how the Centers for Disease Control's messages were coopted by media over the course of the outbreak.

The final part offers a bioethical perspective on the response to the EVD outbreak. In chapter 13, Michael Selgelid—a member of the WHO ethical advisory panel for the use of unregistered interventions in combatting EVD—offers an account of the role of "clinical equipoise" in the ethics of using unregistered interventions in the outbreak. In chapter 14, Annette Rid details the ethical considerations that drove one of the most controversial aspects of the outbreak response: the pursuit of clinical trials of experimental therapies within West Africa during the outbreak. Rid's chapter is complemented with one by Morenike Oluwatoyin Folayan and Bridget Haire, who provide a counterargument against the use of randomized clinical trials in an outbreak zone. The choice to include two chapters on the clinical trials issue was intentional on our part, as the ethics of clinical trials in the context of the EVD outbreak split the scientific, clinical, and bioethical communities. Kelly Hills rounds out the section with a discussion of the ethics of quarantine, which played a significant political role in the response to EVD within the United States.

This volume is completed with an epilogue written by Lisa M. Lee, executive director of the Presidential Commission for the Study of Bioethical Issues. Lee, in her role on the commission, oversaw its inquiry into the ethics of public health responses to disease epidemics in light of the EVD outbreak, the first of many attempts to unpack the outbreak and learn from the mistakes that generated the catastrophe.[5] Lee recounts this process, and how policy-making bodies can apply themselves to building policies around infectious disease that, we hope, will lead to better results in the future.

It is our belief that, in addition to the exceptional content our contributors have imparted, this work is itself an argument in favor of a specific model of scholarship in infectious disease—one that values multidisciplinary collaboration over academic silos. This work should appeal to a wide range of practitioners, researchers, and educators: There is something in here for everyone, and the chapters were written to incorporate into coursework as readings that are complementary to other studies of public health, medicine, and basic science. An examination of the 2013–2016 Ebola outbreak can serve as a microcosm of the larger challenges present in global public health. If Ebola's message can be anything, it is our hope that it will be an invitation to work together.

Notes

1. World Health Organization, "Ebola Situation Report," October 28, 2015, http://apps.who.int/iris/bitstream/10665/191299/1/ebolasitrep_28Oct2015_eng.pdf?ua=1.

2. J. K. Taubenberger and D. M. Morens, "1918 Influenza: The Mother of All Pandemics," *Revista Biomédica* 17 (2006): 69–79.

3. Barry Hewlett and Bonnie Hewlett. *Ebola, Culture and Politics: The Anthropology of an Emerging Disease* (Belmont, CA: Cengage Learning, 2007).

4. J. Knobloch, E. J. Albiez, and H. Schmitz. "A Serological Survey on Viral Haemorrhagic Fevers in Liberia," *Annales De l'Institut Pasteur/Virologie* 133, no. 2 (January 1982): 125–28, doi: 10.1016/S0769-2617(82)80028-2.

5. Lisa M. Lee, *Ethics and Ebola* (Washington, DC: Presidential Commission for the Study of Bioethical Issues, 2015).

1 What Is Ebola?

1 What Is Ebola?

Stephen Goldstein

Since its discovery in 1976, and especially since Richard Preston published *The Hot Zone* in 1994, Ebola has been an evocative word in the American consciousness. A 1995 outbreak in Zaire (now the Democratic Republic of the Congo), reported on extensively by *The New York Times,* cemented the word "Ebola" into the American lexicon. The result: Ebola virus, named after the Ebola River in the Democratic Republic of the Congo, has both frightened and fascinated for decades. Many Americans know the rough outlines: that it is an African virus, that it has killed 50–90 percent of those infected in most outbreaks, that it emerges suddenly from the forest before disappearing again. Its emergence and explosion in West Africa in December 2013 has elevated it from a fascinating curiosity to the front pages and to the front of minds. Along with its high-profile appearance on the global stage have come misunderstanding and fear. These stem from a lack of knowledge—not from lack of interest, but rather from the relative inaccessibility of scientific information. Among these gaps in the public knowledge are what Ebola virus actually is, where it comes from (as best we know), how it causes disease, and how it spreads. We begin with the simplest question of the four: What is Ebola virus?

Taxonomy of Ebolavirus

Viruses represent a vast taxon apart from the recognized kingdoms of life. They are vanishingly small, yet infect every known living organism. Viral taxonomy is a sort of poor man's approximation of taxonomy among the three kingdoms of life. Within the viral universe, Ebola virus fits into a small, poorly understood family of viruses, the *Filoviridae.* The filoviruses fall into three genera within *Filoviridae*: *Ebolavirus*, *Marburgvirus*, and *Cuevavirus*. Of these, *Cuevavirus* is the simplest; its sole constituent virus, *Lloviu virus*, is known only by a genome sequence recovered from dead European bats.[1]

Marburg virus, discovered in 1967, was the first filovirus to be identified and has since caused small, sporadic outbreaks throughout Africa. The genus *Marburgvirus* consists of one viral species, *Marburg marburgvirus*, which consists of two member viruses, Marburg virus and Ravn virus.[2] These two viruses, though slightly different, cause the same clinical disease in infected individuals, as do the ebolaviruses, to which we now turn.

The genus *Ebolavirus* contains five viral species, four of which are known to cause human disease and three of which have caused outbreaks. *Zaire ebolavirus* comprises Ebola virus, the particular virus that has caused the West Africa Ebola epidemic and which has been responsible for the majority of prior human outbreaks as well. The other viruses that cause the same human disease as Ebola virus are Sudan virus (*Sudan ebolavirus* species), Bundibugyo virus (*Bundibugyo ebolavirus* species), and Tai Forest virus (*Tai forest ebolavirus* species); however, these three viruses have thus far been less fatal than *Zaire ebolavirus*.[3] Reston virus, the fifth *Ebolavirus* species, belongs to the species *Reston ebolavirus* and was the subject of *The Hot Zone*, which described a Reston virus outbreak within a Virginia primate holding facility. Reston virus is thought to be nonpathogenic in humans and also the only ebolavirus found outside of Africa. All available epidemiological evidence suggests that it is of Asian origin.

The Elusive Hiding Place of Ebola Virus

One of the troubling aspects of Ebola virus' emergence has been its capacity to cause sporadic outbreaks and disappear back into the forest. After the first recognized outbreak in 1976, the virus vanished for nearly twenty years before reappearing in 1995 in the city of Kikwit, Zaire. The scientists and epidemiologists who led the international response in 1976 prioritized identifying the reservoir host of Ebola virus; they hoped that understanding where the virus came from might aid prevention or prediction of future outbreaks. Despite testing hundreds of animals from dozens of species, they came up empty. Similar work following the 1995 outbreak failed to identify the virus or past evidence of infection in any of the 3,066 animals collected.[4]

In 2005 a research group led by Eric Leroy of the Centre International de Recherches Médicales de Franceville in Gabon finally made a critical discovery. They collected over 1,000 birds, bats, and small terrestrial mammals in the vicinity of an ongoing Ebola outbreak among gorillas and chimpanzees. Among these, individual bats of three species—*Hypsignathus monstrosus, Epomops franqueti* and *Myonycteris torquata*—contained antibodies against Ebola virus, indicating past infection. Other bats of the same three species contained fragments of the Ebola virus genome in their livers and spleens. However, the amount of viral RNA in the samples was very low, and attempts to isolate live Ebola virus from these samples were unsuccessful.[5] Later studies that tested other bat species for previous infection with Ebola virus identified additional possible reservoirs, including *Rousettus aegyptiacus,* a reservoir of Marburg virus.[6,7] The discovery that multiple species of bat might serve as reservoirs greatly complicates the task of predicting and preventing spillovers into the human population.

Although we now know that various bat species are the probable reservoir, there are still important unknowns about the behavior of Ebola virus in its natural host. Some of these questions have implications for the pattern of Ebola virus outbreaks in humans. We don't know, for example, why outbreaks are so rare, or why they occur when they do. It may be that Ebola virus prevalence is very low in the reservoir population but surges intermittently. It is also possible that Ebola virus loads in the natural host are so low that viral shedding by bats is typically minimal, yet viral load may also fluctuate and result in increased likelihood of spillover into humans at certain times. The answer may be as simple as that contact between bats and humans is relatively rare, but becomes more frequent under certain environmental conditions.

Additionally, many Ebola virus outbreaks in humans have occurred concurrently with outbreaks in great apes and some have been associated with human exposure to infected ape carcasses. The dynamics of ape-bat interactions are largely unknown, though their consumption of similar types of fruit provides an obvious opportunity for Ebola virus spillover into primates, and the existence of an intermediate host increases the complexity of preventing spillover into humans.

Ebola Virus Structure and Genome

Everything a virus does to promote its own replication and transmission to a new host is driven by its structure and the functions of the proteins encoded by its genome. Ebola virus consists of a protein-coated genome, matrix proteins that support the structure of the virion, or single virus particle, and a lipid envelope that is co-opted from the host-cell membrane when new virions exit the host cell. Together, these factors give Ebola virus and other filoviruses a distinctive thread-like appearance that is strikingly different than that of other known viruses.

Unlike animals, plants, and bacteria, which all use DNA to store genetic information, viruses may use DNA or RNA. DNA viruses include herpesviruses and poxviruses while RNA viruses include influenza viruses, flaviviruses like West Nile virus, and the filoviruses. The RNA viruses are further classified by the organization of their genome, and by how many steps are required to make proteins encoded by their RNA.

The simplest distinction is between positive and negative-sense viral RNA genomes. Positive-sense RNA genomes, such as that of West Nile virus, are essentially viral versions of our own protein-coding messenger RNAs (mRNA); both can be directly translated into proteins by host-cell ribosomes. Often, the proteins of viruses with positive-sense RNA genomes are translated as one or two large polyproteins that are then cleaved into individual proteins.

Negative-sense RNA genomes differ significantly in that they cannot be directly translated into protein. Rather, they must be transcribed into full-length positive-sense RNA anti-genomes to begin genome replication and smaller viral mRNAs as the first step in protein synthesis. Either of these can then be translated into protein by the host protein synthesis machinery. Some RNA genomes exist in multiple pieces, such as the negative-sense segmented RNA genome of influenza virus. Most, however—including filovirus genomes—are a single strand of RNA.

Ebola virus has a 19 kilobase-long negative-sense RNA genome containing seven genes, which encode eight proteins. The nucleoprotein (NP), VP30, and VP35 proteins comprise the protein component of the nucleocapsid complex, the assembly of proteins that tightly coats the viral genomic RNA.[8] The major component of this complex is NP, which forms a helical structure that surrounds the viral genome. The L protein is the viral

RNA-dependent RNA-polymerase, the enzyme required for transcribing positive-sense copies of the viral genome and transcribing viral mRNAs.

The glycoprotein (GP) is the primary viral surface protein; it is sugar-coated and mediates attachment to the cellular receptor and subsequent entry into the host cell. After GP is made, three different GP molecules associate with each other to form a trimer. This trimer is then coated in sugars, or glycosolated, and is incorporated into the viral envelope, and will ultimately play a critical role in Ebola virus entry into a host cell.

In addition to GP, which is anchored to the surface of the Ebola virion and sticks outward, Ebola virus also produces a soluble version of GP (sGP) that is secreted from infected cells. Though the other Ebola virus proteins are similar structurally and functionally to those produced by Marburg virus, synthesis of sGP is unique to Ebola virus. Soluble GP likely serves a role in immune evasion, specifically in rendering the host antibody response ineffective. Though its role was poorly understood for years, recent evidence suggests sGP induces the host to produce antibodies that will bind itself in addition to full-length GP.[9] As a result, sGP effectively soaks up antibodies that might otherwise bind full-length GP and neutralize the virus. Indeed, this role is seemingly so important that Ebola virus actually produces more sGP than full-length GP.

VP40 is the matrix protein that provides structure to virions and lies just under the lipid envelope that the virus steals from its host as it exits the cell.[10] VP24 is a poorly understood minor matrix protein that plays a role in assembling the Ebola nucleocapsid complex and also is active in disrupting the host response to infection.[11]

Through the activity of these different proteins, Ebola virus is able to infect and replicate to tremendous levels inside a host, prevent an effective immune response, and—in the case of primates—cause a devastating disease. All of this requires an initial, complex step mediated by GP: entry into a host-cell.

Ebola Virus Host Cell Entry

Viruses as a rule lack the ability to replicate on their own; thus, they must co-opt host cell machinery to replicate and produce new virus particles. For any virus, and Ebola virus is no exception, the first step to replication is entry into a susceptible host cell. Virus entry into a host cell is a multistep process involving both viral and host proteins. Most enveloped viruses enter cells via receptor-mediated endocytosis, which begins after the viral glycoprotein attaches in a highly specific fashion to a receptor molecule on the surface of the host cell. After attachment, the receptor and virus are brought into the cell inside an endosome, which is an acidic vesicle containing enzymes required for the glycoprotein to facilitate exit from the endosome. The virion will effectively disassemble in the endosome, allowing its protein-coated genome to enter the cytoplasm of the host cell, where its replication cycle can begin.

Ebola virus, which is unusually large, uses a somewhat unusual pathway to enter host cells, and identifying its receptor was a challenge not overcome until 2011.[12] Rather than entering cells by surface receptor-mediated endocytosis like most enveloped viruses, Ebola virus and other filoviruses enter cells via a process called macropinocytosis, which does not require a specific cell-surface receptor (unlike, say, influenza).[13] Rather, macropinocytosis occurs when cell-surface molecules like DC-SIGN or TIM-1,[14] which have been identified as Ebola virus entry factors, recognize a large molecule, or in this case, a virion, in the space outside the cell. In the case of Ebola virus, these cell-surface molecules likely recognize host cell-derived molecules on the viral envelope called phosphatidylserines. Ultimately Ebola virus ends up in the same place, an acidified endosome, as other viruses; it just takes a slightly different route in getting there.

Although DC-SIGN and TIM-1 are known Ebola virus entry factors, they do not appear to be strictly required for entry.[15] Rather, a cellular cholesterol transport protein, NPC-1, serves as the actual entry receptor inside the endosome.[16] After binding NPC-1, the Ebola virus GP trimer is cleaved by specialized enzymes, called proteases, in the endosome causing GP to change its shape, or undergo a conformational change. This conformational change causes GP to insert into the endosomal membrane, causing a fusion of the viral envelope and the endosomal membrane. This fusion facilitates delivery of the Ebola virus genome, wrapped tightly in a protein coat, into the host cell cytoplasm, where the rest of its life cycle proceeds.

Ebola Virus Replication

After uncoating of the genome in the host-cell cytoplasm, Ebola virus initiates two distinct processes to produce new viral particles. It must both replicate its genome and manipulate the host cell into synthesizing the eight viral proteins. Replication of the genome occurs in two steps, involving both viral and host-cell proteins.

The principal viral protein involved is the L protein, the RNA-dependent RNA-polymerase (RdRp) that each Ebola virion carries into a host cell. Ebola and other RNA viruses must encode an RdRp in their own genomes because host-cell polymerases will only use DNA templates to make RNA, whereas the virus provides an RNA template. The viral polymerase, L in the case of Ebola virus, makes a positive-sense copy of the negative-sense RNA genome. This copy, or anti-genome, serves as a template for L to make a new negative-sense genome (in the same way a negative image can be used to create a copy of a photograph). Multiple host proteins participate in this process as well, likely in the role of stabilizing the RNA-polymerase complex and making sure the viral genome is in a configuration that allows it to be transcribed by L.

Viral protein synthesis, or translation, also requires significant involvement of viral and host proteins. Specifically, viruses lack any ability to synthesize their own proteins, and so both nucleic acid and protein components of the host protein synthesis machinery are essential for the viral life cycle. The first step in viral protein synthesis is L transcribing each of the seven Ebola virus genes into positive-sense viral mRNA, which can be recognized by the host protein translation machinery. Sometimes a less than full length mRNA is made from the GP gene, and synthesis of sGP is the result. Following transcription, the viral mRNAs are modified at each end so the host translation machinery can recognize them.

After a new genome has been produced and the viral proteins synthesized, the RNA and proteins need to assemble into new virions that can leave the cell that produced them and find new targets. The first step in this process is the formation of the nucleocapsid, the RNA-protein complex that comprises the structural core of the virion. NP, by now the most abundant protein in the entire cell, is the key player in this complex. It tightly wraps newly transcribed Ebola virus genomes and is the scaffold for formation of the nucleocapsid that also includes VP35, VP40, VP24, and L. The nucleocapsid has an elongated, helical structure that provides the distinctive shape of an Ebola virion. The nucleocapsid is transported to the cell membrane, where GP awaits. The virion then buds from the cell, stealing some of the cell membrane with GP incorporated in it as it leaves.

Overall, viral replication is so efficient and robust that viral RNA may ultimately become the most abundant RNA in a host cell and viral proteins the most abundant proteins. Over time, a single Ebola virus particle will turn a cell into a virus-producing factory that is able to pump out millions of new virions before it dies. Ultimately, an infected cell may be recognized and killed by host immune cells, or may die due to the relentless production of new virions, each of which steals a piece of the cell membrane on its way out. Exactly what happens to an infected cell is irrelevant to the virus as long as it lives long enough to propagate the infection. The same is true on a larger scale regarding transmission of Ebola virus, a topic that has become particularly fraught over the course of the ongoing epidemic.

Ebola Virus Transmission

Two great misconceptions predominate the public discourse on Ebola. The first is that patients bleed to death; in fact, the percentage of cases with hemorrhaging is much lower than observed for other symptoms. By a large margin the most common symptoms of EVD are fever, malaise, diarrhea, abdominal pain, and vomiting, which are observed in 55–90 percent of patients.[17] Hemorrhagic symptoms are observed less frequently and are not necessarily correlated with a fatal outcome. In a large 2014 Sierra Leone study, only 1 of 106 patients exhibited signs of hemorrhage,[18] while 19 out of 37 patients experienced some bleeding in a contemporaneous study in Guinea.[19] During the 1995 Kikwit outbreak, up to 50 percent of patients exhibited some hemorrhagic symptoms.[20, 21] While these data suggest that different variants even within an outbreak may be more or less likely to cause hemorrhage, most hemorrhagic symptoms were minor, such as bleeding gums, bleeding from injection sites, and some blood in vomit or diarrhea rather than massive hemorrhage. Hemorrhage has never been evaluated as a leading cause of death due to Ebola virus disease. Rather, death is primarily due to complications of catastrophic dehydration as a result of fluid loss from vomiting and diarrhea that can exceed 5–10 liters/day, resulting in life-threatening electrolyte deficiencies.

The second misconception, by far the more dangerous, is that Ebola can spread through the air like a cold or influenza. The science on how Ebola virus is transmitted is actually quite clear. Both experimental research in macaques and careful epidemiological work during and after human outbreaks have failed to demonstrate any credible evidence of airborne spread. One widely cited 2012 article showed that Ebola virus might be able to spread through the air between pigs and macaques,[22] but a follow-up study showed that this could not occur between macaques—a much more relevant model for a human outbreak.[23]

The epidemiological data from human outbreaks clearly demonstrates that direct bodily contact or contact with the fluids of a person actually suffering from EVD puts one at the highest risk of transmission.[24] Contact with blood, vomit, and diarrhea of EVD patients carries a high risk of transmission, as may contact with sweat and saliva late in infection.[25] Finally, the current West African epidemic has featured the first documented sexual transmission of Ebola virus in a woman with no risk factors other than having had sex with a survivor. This man's semen tested positive for virus nearly identical to that isolated from the woman.[26]

Historically, people with limited contact with EVD patients, or who only were in contact with infected individuals before the onset of disease, have not become sick themselves. This is almost certainly because virus levels in the blood of infected individuals before symptom onset are very low. Early in infection, the virus is largely confined to the liver and the spleen, where it replicates vigorously and causes tremendous damage. Virus only becomes reliably detectable in the blood two to three days after infection, which is when the risk of transmission begins to rise.[27] Until then, even people who may ultimately progress to severe EVD and die are extremely unlikely to transmit the virus.

Conclusion

The 2013–2016 West African Ebola epidemic has opened the world's eyes to what had—until recently—been a frightening but little seen virus. Nevertheless—however terrifying, however (seemingly) unique and horrible the disease—Ebola is bound by the same rules and made of the same kinds of molecules as any other virus. Through a basic understanding of the science underlying Ebola virus we might beat back the fear that has coursed through West Africa and around the world, move toward better, science-based public health policy, and build a framework for responding more rapidly, comprehensively, and effectively to the next epidemic.

Notes

1. Ana Negredo, Gustavo Palacios, Sonia Vázquez-Morón, Félix González, Hernán Dopazo, Francisca Molero, et al., "Discovery of an Ebolavirus-Like Filovirus in Europe," *PLoS Pathogens* 7, no. 10 (October 2011), doi: e1002304.

2. Jens H. Kuhn, Stephan Becker, Hideki Ebihara, Thomas W. Geisbert, Karl M. Johnson, Yoshihiro Kawaoka, et al., "Proposal for a Revised Taxonomy of the Family *Filoviridae*: Classification, Names of Taxa and Viruses, and Virus Abbreviations," *Archives of Virology* 155, no. 12 (December 2010): 2083–2103.

3. Ibid.

4. Herwig Leirs, James N. Mills, John W. Krebs, James E. Childs, Dudu Akaibe, Neal Woollen, et al., "Search for the Ebola Virus Reservoir in Kikwit, Democratic Republic of the Congo: Reflections on a Vertebrate Collection," *Journal of Infectious Diseases* 179, no. 1 (February 1999): S155–63.

5. Eric M. Leroy, Brice Kumulungui, Xavier Pourrut, Pierre Rouquet, Alexandre Hassanin, Philippe Yaba, et al., "Fruit Bats as Reservoirs of Ebola Virus," *Nature* 438, no. 7068 (December 1, 2005): 575–76.

6. Xavier Pourrut, Marc Souris, Jonathan S Towner, Pierre E Rollin, Stuart T Nichol, Jean-Paul Gonzalez, et al., "Large Serological Survey Showing Cocirculation of Ebola and Marburg Viruses in Gabonese Bat Populations, and a High Seroprevalence of Both Viruses in Rousettus Aegyptiacus," *BMC Infectious Diseases* 9, no. 1 (2009): 159–168.

7. Xavier Pourrut, André Délicat, Pierre E. Rollin, Thomas. G. Ksiazek, Jean-Paul Gonzalez, and Eric M. Leroy, "Spatial and Temporal Patterns of Zaire Ebolavirus Antibody Prevalence in the Possible Reservoir Bat Species," *Journal of Infectious Diseases* 196, no. 2 (November 15, 2007): S176–83.

8. Viktor E. Volchkov, Valentina A. Volchkova, Elke Muhlberger, Larissa V. Kolesnikova, Michael Weik, Olga Dolnik, et al., "Recovery of Infectious Ebola Virus from Complementary DNA: RNA Editing of the GP Gene and Viral Cytotoxicity," *Science* 291, no. 5510 (March 9, 2001): 1965–69.

9. Gopi S. Mohan, Wenfang Li, Ling Ye, Richard W. Compans, and Chinglai Yang, "Antigenic Subversion: A Novel Mechanism of Host Immune Evasion by Ebola Virus." *PLoS Pathogens* 8, no. 12 (2012): e1003065.

10. Steven Theriault, Allison Groseth, Gabriele Neumann, Yoshihiro Kawaoka, Heinz Feldmann, "Rescue of Ebola Virus From cDNA Using Heterologous Support Proteins," *Virus Research* 106, no. 1 (November 2004): 43–50.

11. Yue Huang, Ling Xu, Yongnian Sun, and Gary J. Nabel, "The Assembly of Ebola Virus Nucleocapsid Requires Virion-Associated Proteins 35 and 24 and

Posttranslational Modification of Nucleoprotein," *Molecular Cell* 10, no. 2 (August 2002): 307–16.

12. Jan E. Carette, Matthijs Raaben, Anthony C. Wong, Andrew S. Herbert, Gregor Obernosterer, Nirupama Mulherkar, et al., "Ebola Virus Entry Requires the Cholesterol Transporter Niemann-Pick C1," *Nature* 477, no. 7364 (September 15, 2011): 340–43.

13. Paulina Aleksandrowicz, Andrea Marzi, Nadine Biedenkopf, Nadine Beimforde, Stephan Becker, Thomas Hoenen, et al., "Ebola Virus Enters Host Cells by Macropinocytosis and Clathrin-Mediated Endocytosis," *Journal of Infectious Diseases* 204, no. 3 (November 2011): S957–67.

14. Andrew S. Kondratowicz, Nicholas J. Lennemann, Patrick L. Sinn, Robert A. Davey, Catherine L. Hunt, Sven Moller-Tank, et al., "T-Cell Immunoglobulin and Mucin Domain 1 (TIM-1) Is a Receptor for Zaire Ebolavirus and Lake Victoria Marburgvirus," *Proceedings of the National Academy of Sciences* 108, no. 20 (May 17, 2011): 8426–31.

15. Carmen P. Alvarez, Fátima Lasala, Jaime Carrillo, Oscar Muñiz, Angel L. Corbí, and Rafael Delgado, "C-Type Lectins DC-SIGN and L-SIGN Mediate Cellular Entry by Ebola Virus in Cis and in Trans," *Journal of Virology* 76, no. 13 (2002): 6841–6844.

16. Carette et al., "Ebola Virus Entry Requires the Cholesterol Transporter Niemann-Pick C1."

17. Mpia A. Bwaka, Marie-José Bonnet, Philippe Calain, Robert Colebunders, Ann De Roo, Yves Guimard, et al., "Ebola Hemorrhagic Fever in Kikwit, Democratic Republic of the Congo: Clinical Observations in 103 Patients," *Journal of Infectious Diseases* 179 (January 15, 1999): S1–S7.

18. John S. Schieffelin, Jeffrey G. Shaffer, Augustine Goba, Michael Gbakie, Stephen K. Gire, Andres Colubri, et al., "Clinical Illness and Outcomes in Patients with Ebola in Sierra Leone," *New England Journal of Medicine* 371, no. 22 (November 27, 2014): 2092–2100.

19. Elhadj Ibrahima Bah, Marie-Claire Lamah, Tom Fletcher, Shevin T. Jacob, David M. Brett-Major, Amadou Alpha Sall, et al., "Clinical Presentation of Patients with Ebola Virus Disease in Conakry, Guinea," *New England Journal of Medicine* 372, no. 1 (January 1, 2015): 40–47.

20. Bwaka et al., "Ebola Hemorrhagic Fever in Kikwit, Democratic Republic of the Congo: Clinical Observations in 103 Patients."

21. Roger Ndambi, Philippe Akamituna, Marie-Jo Bonnet, Anicet Mazaya Tukadila, Jean-Jacques Muyembe-Tamfum, and Robert Colebunders, "Epidemiologic and Clinical Aspects of the Ebola Virus Epidemic in Mosango, Democratic Republic of the Congo, 1995," *Journal of Infectious Diseases* 179 (January 15, 1999): S8–S10.

22. Hana M. Weingartl, Carissa Embury-Hyatt, Charles Nfon, Anders Leung, Greg Smith, and Gary Kobinger, "Transmission of Ebola Virus from Pigs to Non-Human Primates," *Scientific Reports* 2 (November 15, 2012).

23. Judie Alimonti, Anders Leung, Shane Jones, Jason Gren, Xiangguo Qiu, Lisa Fernando, et al., "Evaluation of Transmission Risks Associated with In Vivo Replication of Several High Containment Pathogens in a Biosafety Level 4 Laboratory," *Scientific Reports* 4 (July 25, 2014).

24. Scott F. Dowell, Rose Mukunu, Thomas G. Ksiazek, Ali S. Khan, Pierre E. Rollin, and C. J. Peters, "Transmission of Ebola Hemorrhagic Fever: A Study of Risk Factors in Family Members, Kikwit, Democratic Republic of the Congo, 1995," *Journal of Infectious Diseases* 179 (January 15, 1999): S87–S91.

25. Paolo Francesconi, Zabulon Yoti, Silvia Declich, Paul Awil Onek, Massimo Fabiani, Joseph Olango, et al., "Ebola Hemorrhagic Fever Transmission and Risk Factors of Contacts, Uganda," *Emerging Infectious Diseases* 9, no. 11 (October 21, 2003): 1430–37.

26. Athalia Christie, Gloria J. Davies-Wayne, Thierry Cordier-Lasalle, David J. Blackley, A. Scott Laney, Desmond E. Williams, et al., "Possible Sexual Transmission of Ebola Virus—Liberia, 2015," *MMWR. Morbidity and Mortality Weekly Report* 64, no. 17 (May 8, 2015): 479–81.

27. Jonathan S. Towner, Pierre E. Rollin, Daniel G. Bausch, Anthony Sanchez, Sharon M. Crary, Martin Vincent, et al., "Rapid Diagnosis of Ebola Hemorrhagic Fever by Reverse Transcription-PCR in an Outbreak Setting and Assessment of Patient Viral Load as a Predictor of Outcome," *Journal of Virology* 78, no. 8 (January 15, 2004): 4330–41.

2 Ebola in West Africa: From the Frontline

Patricia C. Henwood

From the frontlines in West Africa, there are a variety of lessons to be learned when evaluating the sociological, political, and anthropological factors that contributed to the evolution of the 2013–2016 Ebola virus disease (EVD) epidemic. Additionally, the outbreak provides its share of lessons for the management of EVD in individual patients, as well as the balance between public health needs and clinical medicine. In this chapter, I discuss the challenges facing health care workers (HCWs) during this 2013–2016 epidemic and what can be learned in order to strengthen future global public health responses.

Background

While most previous EVD outbreaks occurred in rural areas, the geography of the 2013–2016 epidemic created multiple challenges. The virus initially presented itself in a forested region, similar to past outbreaks, likely due to contact with a bat vector or consumption of infected bush meat. This forested region encompasses the porous borders of three previously Ebola-naïve West African countries with mobile populations that share a similar ethnic group and language and have accessible roads between their major urban centers.

EVD quickly demonstrated its disrespect for political boundaries within the region, crossing from Guinea into Sierra Leone, Liberia, Nigeria, and Mali within months. The ease of human migration within the region; a combination of both rural areas with limited health care and densely populated capital cities; cross-border politics; and difficulty with coordination made it challenging to initially investigate case leads and maintain effective contact tracing efforts. Additionally, community resistance to containment efforts, fueled by misunderstandings about EVD, negatively impacted case identification and contact tracing efforts.

Traditional burial practices and funeral rights in the region often involve washing and touching the body of the deceased. Safe burials in the context of EVD require extensive protective equipment to prevent disease transmission to family and those caring for the body as bodily fluids of EVD patients are believed to be the most virulent when their bodies are overcome by EVD at the time of death. In the context of the 2013–2016 outbreak, contact with these very infectious bodily fluids often led to numerous new EVD cases and several deaths arising from one traditional burial.

When cases were eventually suspected and identified, the overburdened health care system was limited in its ability to manage cases and control the epidemic. The lack of material resources, such as appropriate personal protective equipment and diagnostic equipment, presented a significant barrier to management. This was compounded by relatively low numbers of HCWs, especially those with training in relevant infection prevention and control principles for EVD. The death of many HCWs early in the course of the epidemic, along with issues with the availability of relevant equipment and appropriate compensation for local HCWs that considered the risks of the work they were assuming, also presented a significant barrier to care.[1]

The World Health Organization (WHO) estimates that in the three most impacted countries—Guinea, Sierra Leone, and Liberia—there are only one to two physicians available to treat 100,000 people.[2] In addition, most of these physicians are concentrated in urban areas, leaving large parts of the country without access to physician services. These countries also have among the lowest numbers of trained nurses and midwives in the world relative to population density.[3] This translates into an unsustainable workload for local health care providers that affects productivity, quality, and job satisfaction, and likely contributes to challenges of emigration or "brain drain" of the trained health care workforce.

The impacted countries had been making improvements in the health sector prior to this EVD outbreak. For example, Liberia had nearly halved its maternal mortality ratio (per 100,000 live births), from 1,200 in 2000 to 640 in 2013.[4] Attempts to better train and retain local talent were underway, and Liberia had increased intake and scope of its postgraduate training programs for physicians just months prior to Ebola's emergence.[5] Despite forward progress, the regional health care infrastructure still proved under-resourced to manage the emergence of this new virus.

Despite being involved with management of the initial outbreak, miscalculations were made by WHO and US Centers for Disease Control (CDC) experts on the trajectory and complexity of this outbreak in the spring of 2014. Meanwhile, EVD was crossing borders in the Kissi language area and traveling through the region largely unrecognized for some time.[6]

Early symptoms of Ebola appear similar to regionally endemic illnesses such as malaria, typhoid, and Lassa fever. Despite decades of prior outbreaks elsewhere on the continent, West Africa had never before documented a case of EVD. Dr. Margaret Chan, director general of the WHO, noted "old diseases in new context will deliver surprises," and these post-conflict countries lacked the trust needed to initially mobilize communities to be part of the solution. Some impacted populations had baseline suspicion of the state, considering prolonged periods during which their basic needs were not provided for after having recently emerged from decades of political coups in Guinea, prolonged civil wars in Sierra Leone and Liberia, and transnational conflicts. Moreover, impacted governments in this fragile post-conflict reconstruction phase had not previously dealt with the unique social and economic disruptions of EVD.

Initial Impact on HCWs

By August 2014, 12 percent of deaths from Ebola in Liberia were among HCWs alone.[7] Historically, HCWs have accounted for up to 25 percent of those infected in previous outbreaks.[8] HCW exposure to EVD is more often in the general hospital or clinic setting and less often in dedicated Ebola treatment centers. This may be the result of unrecognized or mis-triaged cases, hospital overcrowding, and lack of training in or availability of appropriate personal protective equipment and infection control practices. Rising infections and lack of appropriate resources among HCWs in the hospital context degraded confidence in the already limited health care infrastructure. This led to the functional closure of much of the existing health care system in impacted areas while Ebola cases were arising. When Ebola was appropriately recognized, there was ongoing difficulty with the ability to refer and transport patients to treatment units or centers with the proper training and protective equipment to provide Ebola care.

As EVD spread quickly in mobile and urban environments, the ability to isolate patients in Ebola treatment units (ETUs) was quickly overwhelmed. Médecins Sans Frontières historically managed much of the clinical care in the context of prior EVD outbreaks in conjunction with the WHO, CDC, and local ministries of health. However, the pace, geographic spread, and magnitude of this epidemic quickly called for the involvement of other humanitarian and medical relief groups to assist in case management.

There are several strains within the *Ebolavirus* genus (for more information, see chapter 1). Deaths from prior outbreaks of the *Zaire ebolavirus* viral species that appeared in Western Africa were as high as 90 percent.[9] This meant that exposure and mortality risk to the extremely limited numbers of HCWs in the region was of paramount concern early in the epidemic. Considering the infectivity and severity of the virus, significant tension existed between the ability to effectively isolate large numbers of patients to prevent community spread of EVD and the ability to provide high-quality patient care to improve chances of individual survival. The public health priority of breaking chains of transmission through isolation of presumed or confirmed cases and safer burials at times took precedence over comprehensive individual case management. For example, when there were overwhelming ratios of patients to trained health care providers, some treatment centers only provided oral medications and did not assume the risks of intravenous therapy (i.e., exposure of HCWs to the blood of patients or to potential needlesticks).

This lack of adequate human and material resources that would have allowed for focus on improvement of individual patient outcomes from EVD arguably undermined the public health response. Some perceived ETUs not as a place to seek treatment, but as a place people went to die, resulting in reluctance to acknowledge symptoms or seek care for EVD. This resistance potentially led to more deaths and unsafe burials in communities while propagating transmission, especially since traditional funerals often involved unsafe burials (by Ebola management standards) and transmission from dead bodies led to many new Ebola cases.[10]

International Awareness and Response

For the first time in history, an emergency meeting of the United Nations Security Council was called because of the overwhelming nature of the public health crisis. HCWs on the ground in West Africa at the time were relatively few, and those who were present were both overstretched and underresourced in attempting to manage the skyrocketing caseload and infection prevention measures. WHO's Director General deemed this a public health emergency of international concern (PHEIC) on August 8, 2014, at which point there were already 1,779 cases and 961 deaths.

This was only the third-ever declaration of a PHEIC, the two others being the 2009 H1N1 flu pandemic and the 2014 polio resurgence after its near-eradication. The UN Mission for Ebola Emergency Response was subsequently formed as a coordinating body on September 18, 2014. This was the first-ever UN mission dedicated to public health emergency response. The United States and other members of the international community committed resources, including funding, equipment, and military deployments. The response finally began to scale up more appropriately.

As Ebola patients were repatriated to Europe and the United States for further management, the concern in the international community started to rise in a commensurate fashion. When cases developed in the United States among exposed HCWs, concern about possible domestic outbreaks and modes of transmission escalated. Evolving early guidelines and inconsistent messaging from government officials and the media in August and September 2014 led to skepticism among the public regarding advice from government officials and misgivings about returning HCWs. This distrust resulted in fear superseding science in some cases, such as quarantine restrictions on returning HCWs enacted in New York and New Jersey.[11]

Concern about a potential Ebola outbreak in the United States served to hamper the response in West Africa, leading to restrictions on deploying HCWs, either by employers unwilling to release staff for participation as humanitarian responders or due to concern about evolving government restrictions on returning HCWs. One international humanitarian organization lost approximately 25 percent of their potential Ebola responders when quarantine policies were established.[12] International awareness certainly led to an increase in the material and financial resources mobilized, but the sheer lack of HCWs and delays in resource distribution meant that clinical patient management, even for very basic and commonly treatable medical problems, was limited in most clinical settings. For HCWs who were working to rebuild local systems prior to Ebola's emergence and those responding with an awareness of health care delivery in a high-resource setting, including myself as a clinician, this extreme lack of access to care was distressing to witness.

Scale-Up of the West Africa Response

In late September 2014, the Centers for Disease Control released their first Ebola response prediction models. This epidemiologic modeling tool was based on Ebola case data and doubling times for the virus in Liberia and Sierra Leone through late August. The model projected that if the EVD epidemic were to continue without intervention, as of January 20, 2015, cases would be estimated to reach 550,000 (or 1.4 million cases if corrections were made for underreporting). The same prediction models indicated that if intervention were scaled up such that 70 percent of patients were in treatment or isolation, and if there were changes in community behavior, particularly decreases in unsafe burial practices, as of January 20, 2015, there would be 14,000–35,000 cases.[13]

While slow to launch, the support provided to the local health care systems and governments by the international response did allow for further case management, tracing of suspected or confirmed Ebola cases, and social mobilization.

As more treatment centers opened, more staff were trained, and more resources were provided in terms of protective equipment, there was more of an ability to shift from a focus on isolation and minimal treatment to increased intervention and improvement in patient mortality. Reflecting the CDC prediction models, scaled-up intervention helped reduce potential cases by an order of magnitude. Based on the WHO situation reports, cases were at approximately 22,000 as of January 20, 2015. As of September 2, 2015, cases were still within the CDC-predicted range given intervention at approximately 28,073.[14]

Ideally, we would have better systems in place to immediately mobilize the resources necessary so that future responses will not experience tension between isolation for the public good and the highest possible standard of clinical care for the individual patient. For the remainder of this chapter, I'll talk about the deficits in knowledge and care, and what we can do to ensure that we do not lose control of future infectious disease outbreaks through inaction, lack of preparedness, and limited clinical knowledge.

Evolving Science, Sociology, and Standards of Care

Prior to this epidemic, EVD had never been managed in the context of a high-resource health care setting. The opportunity to manage EVD in this new setting, combined with the sheer magnitude of the outbreak in Western Africa, led to a marked increase in knowledge about EVD pathophysiology, clinical management, and the sociologic impact of EVD on affected communities.

Initially, baseline strategies successful at controlling prior Ebola outbreaks were employed. These focused on finding suspected cases as soon as possible and getting them into an ETU. Additional strategies included testing with real-time virus diagnostics in field or regional laboratories, following patient contacts for 21 days in order to identify symptom onset as early as possible, and communication and risk-reduction messaging to impacted communities.

The initial challenges posed by the current epidemic and interactions with communities impacted by EVD unveiled the importance of social mobilization and taking community perceptions into account, especially when addressing EVD in a highly mobile population crossing several national borders in a post-conflict setting.[15] Based on my observations in Liberia, attempting to stop rumors and confusion with simple and clearly communicated health promotions messages about Ebola through radio, television, pamphlets, roadside billboards, community and country leaders, health workers, and survivors appears to have eventually been an important factor in prevention and care-seeking behaviors for those with EVD symptoms. A better understanding of community perceptions, reasons for resistance, funeral and burial practices, eating and living styles, and learning best communication channels eventually allowed for more effective messaging and outreach.

Experiences with the recent outbreak should inform best practices in responding to future EVD outbreaks. Regardless of available resources, attention to providing the best available compassionate care to patients, with a focus on minimizing fear and helping maintain hope and dignity, remains paramount in the ETU setting. Anxiety around Ebola is heightened as a result of the personal protective equipment necessary for safe EVD care. When possible, clinicians making themselves known to patients face-to-face across transparent ETU fencing prior to initiating care in protective equipment can help improve care and communication. Surviving patients serve to mobilize others in the community to seek care if they feel they were well cared for in the ETU setting. And for HCWs with limited resuscitation resources, helping afford a dignified death for patients who would otherwise be alone and incapable of caring for themselves appears to be valuable for both patient and provider.

Children represent a particularly vulnerable population and one that is difficult to best care for in the ETU setting. Unaccompanied minors, or those with discordant EVD testing results from their parents or family, present challenges not only in their medical care but also with their safety, supervision, feeding, and so on. EVD mortality for the under five-year-old population is among the highest, and their acute care is particularly difficult for health care workers who can only spend limited time with them due to the constraints of personal protective equipment. This takes both a physical and emotional toll on HCWs. When safe and feasible, cohorting children with relatives or friends, or engaging EVD survivors to assist in their care, may be strategies worth employing.

If children survive to discharge, another set of challenges arise, as they may often be orphaned or stigmatized when attempting to return to their communities. ETUs and partner organizations, with local government as indicated, are charged with coordinating the safe return of children to their families or placement with relatives or protective custody as needed at the time of discharge. Managing the impact of this EVD epidemic on children will need to be a continuing effort considering the long-term regional disruption to schooling, childhood, and family structures in impacted countries.

The ability to engage families of ETU patients, and for patients to interact with visitors, is important not only for the pediatric population, but for all patients receiving ETU care. Transparent fencing, providing a safe area for visitation (at a distance), and allowing families to be present for burial services when possible can aid in this process. Providing religious or psychosocial support to both patients and families is of particular importance. Counselors, pastors, nurses, community leaders, and others should receive focused EVD psychosocial training in order to best support patients, families, and staff around the challenges of seeking Ebola care, providing care in the ETU setting, and discharge back to the community (whether they be negative for EVD or have attained survivor status). All of the above strategies allow for better communication and more dignified care, and appear to improve treatment-seeking behaviors.

Attempts to improve the standard of care for EVD are ongoing. As the epidemic unfolded in real time, frontline HCWs in ETUs on remote Liberian hilltops were searching data from cases managed in high-resource settings. They consulted with organizational or WHO focal points on specific patient-management topics in order to better treat the next ailing patient in their low-resource treatment center with up-to-date information. Coordination with UN Mission for Ebola Emergency Response and WHO experts allowed for knowledge pooling and resources to consult when particular management challenges arose.

EVD management strategies were largely based on expert opinion at the start of this epidemic. There is still much to be learned from the data collected during patient care at the ETUs across West Africa. An important focus moving forward will be thorough analysis of these findings so as to have evidence-based guidelines in place for patient management in the future. Two areas of focus where we are gaining further understanding about pathophysiology and treatment strategies are among pregnant patients and among those with possible bacterial infections secondary to Ebola.

Ebola and Pregnancy

The perspective on pregnant EVD patients evolved during the course of this epidemic, and, again, should inform future clinical practice. Historical data put maternal death rates upward of 90 percent and, at the time of writing, fetal death in the neonatal period is uniform.[16] As a result of this heightened mortality among pregnant women and nonviable fetuses, nonintervention during pregnancy and delivery had been the standard of care. Like most Ebola management strategies until this epidemic, guidelines were based on very limited numbers, small case series, and expert opinions.

Pregnant patients are at increased baseline risk of contracting Ebola because of their contact with health care services for both prenatal and delivery care. Transmission in maternity settings has been an issue in previous major outbreaks. Consequently, in the context of an EVD outbreak, it was challenging for pregnant women to gain access to lifesaving maternal and newborn interventions provided at health facilities. This lack of care caused adverse maternal and neonatal outcomes such as infection or death, regardless of the underlying issue. Increased community outreach and distribution programs for clean delivery kits were vital considering the scale of the epidemic and its secondary impact on the obstetric population.

EVD often causes spontaneous abortion (miscarriage) with heavy bleeding during the first or second trimester. However, unrelated to EVD, spontaneous abortions are the most common complication of early pregnancy and happen to 15 percent of otherwise healthy women in early pregnancy.[17] Therefore, in the setting of an EVD outbreak, common presentations or complications of pregnancy may become suspect EVD cases. This leads to the challenges of care in the more limited context of an ETU, without surgical or procedural capacity, and most often without a blood bank for transfusions as needed for hemorrhage. Alternatively, women may not even seek care in the hospital setting due to fear of getting infected while there.

The overall number of pregnant women impacted in the course of this epidemic remains unknown. It was previously unclear whether EVD transmission from mother to baby was happening during pregnancy, or via exposure in the birth canal, breastfeeding, or simply close contact after birth. Several cases have now confirmed transmission of EVD across the placenta; therefore, even when maternal virus is cleared from the blood, ongoing fetal EVD infection may still imply unique risks at delivery. EVD case reports have recently been published on maternal assistance during delivery contrary to prior recommendations, including amniocentesis, episiotomy, and other procedures done in the maternal healing phase.[18] Good outcomes for these patients have opened the door to more focus on interventions to improve mortality among pregnant EVD patients over the course of the epidemic.

Médecins Sans Frontières opened a dedicated 33-bed maternity unit at one of their Ebola treatment centers in late January 2015 in Sierra Leone in order to provide more specialized care to this impacted population. Since relatively little is known about Ebola and pregnancy, looking at cases and dedicated obstetric management in this unit, along with pooled data from other treatment centers, will help the humanitarian and research communities glean a better understanding of how to treat these vulnerable women and neonates moving forward.

Secondary Infections

Secondary infections are significant risks for patients with EVD; anti-malarial treatment was given empirically in many ETUs from the beginning of the outbreak due to the endemic nature of malaria and overlapping presenting symptoms. EVD is caused by a virus and is thus not responsive to antibiotics that are used to treat bacterial infections. Therefore, antibiotic administration was variable in the ETU setting and, if given, often varied in type, route of administration, timing of initiation, and duration.

There is, however, increasing recognition that secondary bacterial infections may play a larger role than previously assumed. Data from patients treated in higher-resource settings with careful monitoring of their electrolytes (which impact cardiac, neurologic and multi-organ system function) have given insight and informed protocol development for patients in the lower-resource ETU setting. These data have also confirmed several cases of a particular type of bloodstream infection from gram-negative bacteria, confirmed by blood cultures of patients treated in a high-resource setting, which indicate the need for aggressive intravenous antibiotic therapy.[19–21] This is thought to originate from severe gastrointestinal tract manifestations in which bacteria that normally live inside the bowel translocate outside it and cause systemic infections.[22] As a result, many more ETUs provided empiric intravenous antibiotic therapy aimed at bowel pathogens later in the epidemic than initially.

Changes in medical management such as treatment with intravenous antibiotics for possible secondary bacterial infections, electrolyte repletion protocols, and more aggressive critical care measures are the result of the science and understanding of Ebola's pathophysiology evolving in real time. This, combined with more human and material resources available to treat patients later in the course of the epidemic, likely contributed to an apparent reduced fatality rate over the course of the epidemic, observed from the ETU. While supportive care currently remains the keystone of EVD treatment, there are several experimental vaccines, treatments, and point-of-care tests being studied.

Moving Forward

While the 2013–2016 EVD epidemic has ended, continued vigilance and clear community messaging is necessary in order to facilitate early recognition of potential EVD case flare-ups that may continue. Just as important, the international community needs to ensure the rapid evaluation and dissemination of data collected and knowledge gained about EVD transmission patterns, pathophysiology, and clinical management over the course of this epidemic. If an effective vaccine and curative treatments are still lacking, this information will be incredibly useful not only to end this epidemic, but for whenever and wherever the next outbreak occurs, which should be anticipated in the context of animal reservoirs of EVD.

An ongoing commitment to health systems strengthening is also needed for the region to recover from the cascading impact of Ebola. The challenge of access to basic health care, which was marginal but improving prior to the ongoing Ebola outbreak, has been exacerbated by further losses among the HCW population due to EVD. The limited HCW population further aggravates the baseline challenge of stressful conditions of service, and without commensurate recognition and compensation, may lead to emigration for some of the most talented from the pool of HCWs.[23] Therefore, increasing numbers, capacity, diagnostics, treatments, and other material resources needed for the health care workforce to accomplish their jobs is an area that will require significant ongoing investment by the international community, in partnership with local governments and nongovernmental organizations. In addition, assisting severely impacted communities and orphaned children while addressing survivors suffering from stigmatization and post-EVD medical problems—as well as loss of employment, housing, possessions, and family—are all matters of ongoing concern.

The insufficient baseline infrastructure to contain and manage this EVD epidemic in West Africa highlights the role of infectious diseases and epidemics from a national and international security perspective. Ebola has demonstrated that in our interconnected global community, outbreaks can now move faster than the methods historically used to control them. This demands new approaches to the identification, communication, control, and treatment of infectious outbreaks such as EVD in resource-limited settings and offers a new perspective on the importance of health systems strengthening for the global health security agenda.

Notes

1. Will Pooley, "Ebola: Perspectives from a Nurse and Patient," *American Journal of Tropical Medicine and Hygiene* 92 (2015): 223–4, doi: 10.4269/ajtmh.14-0762.

2. World Health Organization, "Ebola Situation Assessment: Unprecedented Number of Medical Staff Infected with Ebola," August 25, 2014, http://www.who.int/mediacentre/news/ebola/25-august-2014/en/.

3. Yohannes Kinfu, Mario R. Dal Poz, Hugo Mercer, and David B. Evans, "The Health Worker Shortage in Africa: Are Enough Physicians and Nurses Being Trained?," *Bulletin of the World Health Organization* 87 (May 2009): 225–30, http://www.who.int/bulletin/volumes/87/3/08-051599-table-T2.html.

4. World Health Organization, "Liberia," accessed May 10, 2015, http://www.who.int/countries/lbr/en/.

5. Patricia McQuilkin, Roseda E. Marshall, Michelle Niescierenko, Venée N. Tubman, Bradley G. Olson, Donna Staton, et al., "A Successful US Academic Collaborative Supporting Medical Education in a Postconflict Setting," *Global Pediatric Health* 1 (2015), 1–7, doi: 10.1177/2333794X14563383.

6. Kevin Sack, Sheri Fink, Pam Belluck, and Adam Nossiter, "How Ebola Roared Back," *The New York Times*, December 29, 2014, http://www.nytimes.com/2014/12/30/health/how-ebola-roared-back.html.

7. Almea Matanock, M. Allison Arwady, Patrick Ayscue, Joseph D. Forrester, Bethany Gaddis, Jennifer C. Hunter, et al. "Ebola Virus Disease Cases among Health Care Workers Not Working in Ebola Treatment Units—Liberia, June–August, 2014," *Morbidity and Mortality Weekly Report* 63 (Early Release, November 14, 2014): 1–5, http://www.cdc.gov/mmwr/preview/mmwrhtml/mm63e1114a3.htm.

8. AM Casillas, AM Nyamathi, A Sosa, CL Wilder, and H Sands. "A Current Review of Ebola Virus: Pathogenesis, Clinical Presentation, and Diagnostic Assessment." *Biological Research For Nursing* 4 (2003): 268–75.

9. World Health Organization, "Ebola Virus Disease," accessed May 30, 2015, http://www.who.int/mediacentre/factsheets/fs103/en/.

10. World Health Organization, "Ebola Situation Report," November 26, 2014, http://apps.who.int/ebola/en/ebola-situation-report/situation-reports/ebola-situation-report-26-november-2014.

11. Matt Flegenheimer, Michael D. Shear, and Michael Barbado, "Under Pressure, Cuomo Says Ebola Quarantines Can Be Spent at Home," *The New York Times,* October 26, 2014, http://www.nytimes.com/2014/10/27/nyregion/ebola-quarantine .html.

12. Margaret Traub, Head of Global Initiatives, International Medical Corps, email message to author, March 18, 2015.

13. Martin I. Meltzer, Charisma Y. Atkins, Scott Santibanez, Barbara Knust, Brett W. Petersen, Elizabeth D. Ervin, et al., "Estimating the Future Number of Cases in the Ebola Epidemic—Liberia and Sierra Leone, 2014–2015," *Morbidity and Mortality Weekly Report* 63 (03, September 26, 2014): 1–14, http://www.cdc.gov/mmwr/ preview/mmwrhtml/su6303a1.htm?s_cid=su6303a1_w.

14. World Health Organization, "Ebola Situation Report," September 2, 2015, http://apps.who.int/ebola/current-situation/ebola-situation-report-2-september -2015.

15. United Nations Development Program, "Assessing the Socio-economic Impacts of Ebola Virus Disease in Guinea, Liberia and Sierra Leone—The Road to Recovery," December 2014, http://www.africa.undp.org/content/dam/rba/docs/Reports/EVD %20Synthesis%20Report%2023Dec2014.pdf.

16. Kibadi Mupapa, Woliere Mukundu, Mpia Ado Bwaka, Mungala Kipasa, Ann De Roo, Kivudi Kuvula, et al. "Ebola Hemorrhagic Fever and Pregnancy," *Journal of Infectious Diseases* 179 (1999): S11–2.

17. "Early Pregnancy Loss: FAQ 090," The American College of Obstetricians and Gynecologists, 2013, accessed May 30, 2015, http://www.acog.org/-/media/ For-Patients/faq090.pdf?dmc=1&ts=20150531T1238214430.

18. F. M. Baggi, A. Taybi, A. Kurth, M. Van Herp, A. Di Caro, and R. Wölfel, et al., "Management of Pregnant Women Infected with Ebola Virus in a Treatment Centre in Guinea, June 2014," *Euro Surveillance* 19 (June 2014): pii=20983, http://www .eurosurveillance.org/images/dynamic/EE/V19N49/art20983.pdf.

19. Diamantis Plachouras, Dominique L. Monnet, and Mike Catchpole, "Severe Ebola Virus Infection Complicated by Gram-Negative Septicemia," *The New England Journal of Medicine* 372 (2015): 1376–7, doi: 10.1056/NEJMc1500455.

20. Benno Kreuels, Dominic Wichmann, Petra Emmerich, Jonas Schmidt-Chanasit, Geraldine de Heer, Stefan Kluge, et al., "A Case of Severe Ebola Virus Infection Complicated by Gram-Negative Septicemia," *The New England Journal of Medicine* 371 (2014): 2394–2401, doi: 10.1056/NEJMoa1411677.

21. Timo Wolf, Gerrit Kann, Stephan Becker, Christoph Stephan, Hans-Reinhardt Brodt, Philipp de Leuw, et al., "Severe Ebola Virus Disease with Vascular Leakage and

Multiorgan Failure: Treatment of a Patient in Intensive Care," *The Lancet* 385 (2015): 1428–35, doi: http://dx.doi.org/10.1016/S0140-6736(14)62384-9.

22. US Department of Health and Human Services and US Centers for Disease Control and Prevention, "Preparing Health care Workers to Work in Ebola Treatment Units in Africa: Training Toolkit," accessed April 16, 2015, http://www.cdc.gov/vhf/ebola/hcp/safety-training-course/training-toolkit.html.

23. Gerardo Chowell and Hiroshi Nishiura, "Transmission Dynamics and Control of Ebola Virus Disease (EVD): A Review," *BioMed Central Medicine* 12 (2014): 196, doi: 10.1186/s12916-014-0196-0.

3 Clinical Management of Ebola Virus Disease in Resource-Rich Settings

Michael J. Connor, Jr.

Ebola virus disease (EVD) was first identified in humans in 1976 and was quickly recognized to be a highly contagious illness with a high fatality rate during multiple small and sporadic outbreaks, which arose in remote, isolated villages primarily in central Africa through 2012. The disease was known to cause marked gastrointestinal symptoms with profound watery diarrhea, electrolyte abnormalities, occasional bleeding, and organ failure leading to death in 60–90 percent of patients. EVD is caused by any one of several subtypes of *ebolavirus* (with the most common causative agent being Zaire Ebola virus, or EBOV) in the family *filovidirae,* along with Marburg virus—a viral pathogen with similar presenting symptoms and fatality rates.[1]

The 2013–2016 West African Ebola outbreak is by far the largest and most complex outbreak of EVD in history. It is the first to spread in large population centers (including national capitals) as well as abroad via air travel. It is believed that this outbreak began in December 2013 with a child in Guinea. From this index case, EVD spread rapidly in Guinea and to neighboring Sierra Leone and Liberia—fueled by poverty, poor national health care infrastructures, suboptimal sanitation and waste disposal, and local customs (especially surrounding death) that exposed many community members to EBOV during burial rituals, which can persist for many days on corpses of those who have died from EVD. Given the slow initial pace of the international governmental response to the accelerating outbreak, distant spread by air travel to other countries in Africa (e.g., Nigeria, Mali) as well as resource-rich settings like the United States seemed unavoidable. Furthermore, as the global response accelerated, there was a dramatic rise of health care workers (HCWs) from other continents traveling to provide medical assistance, including direct patient care throughout the affected region. Almost inevitably, numerous HCWs developed EVD and were evacuated by their governments to their home countries.

The first cases of EVD in resource-rich settings arrived via medical evacuation of two HCWs to Emory University Hospital (EUH) in Atlanta, Georgia, in early August 2014, which were followed shortly by other HCWs who were evacuated to Spain, the United Kingdom, France, Germany, and Italy. As of October 2, 2015, there have been nearly 30 known cases of EVD managed in North America and Europe to date and a total of 28,412 cases and 11,296 deaths globally as a result of the ongoing outbreak.[2]

This chapter will focus on the clinical management of EVD in resource-rich settings and the lessons learned and applied in managing EVD. Moving forward, understanding the lessons and implications of EVD management in resource-rich settings will hopefully provide a model for governments, public health agencies, hospital, and clinicians to develop robust global infrastructures to better respond to future outbreaks and pandemics of other transmissible high-risk infections.

Preparation

There are few centers in the United States and Western Europe equipped to care for highly infectious illnesses under strict biocontainment isolation protocols. Under contract from the US Centers for Disease Control and Prevention, EUH has long maintained, operated, and staffed one such facility. The design of a biocontainment facility and the unique challenges to patient care and protocols have been developed and published in the past,[3] but these biocontainment facilities and procedures have rarely been tested and challenged previously, except during the 2002–2003 SARS outbreak. Furthermore, the challenges of maintaining staffing and biocontainment skills training for such a facility, which had only been very rarely used throughout its existence, cannot be understated.

As EUH and other hospitals became aware that they would be receiving evacuated individuals with EVD, preparations to receive patients had to be accelerated. These preparations included refreshing skills for facility staff still employed at each center, as well as identifying and training new clinical staff—namely, subspecialty physicians (e.g., critical care, anesthesia, etc.) and additional nurses and ancillary staff to provide appropriate staffing levels to care for multiple concurrent patients. Published protocols and guidelines served as the basis for the local protocols at EUH.[4]

While the basics of EVD and its clinical course have been widely described from the current and prior outbreaks,[5] few HCWs at these biocontainment facilities (and none at EUH) had direct firsthand experience of EVD management. As a result, collaboration between national and international experts was necessary to develop the capacity to treat patients with EVD. Furthermore, given the inadequate development of national health care resources in Guinea, Sierra Leone, and Liberia and the isolated nature of prior outbreaks, little was known about the spectrum of clinical phenotypes of EVD beyond the described high fevers, gastroenteritis with brisk vomiting and diarrhea, hepatitis, encephalopathy (i.e., confusion and lethargy), and occasional hemorrhage.

Like most viral illnesses, it was assumed that patients would present with a range of symptoms and severity. However, no publications had described this range of symptoms prior to the arrival of the first evacuated HCWs with EVD. As facilities prepared to care for EVD evacuees in resource-rich settings, many clinical teams were uncertain of the full spectrum of clinical needs these patients would require. Would the patients require advanced life support interventions such as mechanical ventilation for respiratory failure, vasopressors for shock, or renal replacement therapies (i.e., hemodialysis) for acute kidney failure? Could such therapies be provided in an isolation environment? From personal communications with clinicians who initially responded to the outbreak in West Africa, all reported an absence of respiratory manifestations, but would this be the case in resource-rich settings? At a minimum, biocontainment centers around the world were inexperienced at providing advanced life support therapies (e.g., mechanical ventilation, hemodialysis, invasive procedures) in isolation. Ultimately, despite attempts to prepare, when challenged with critically ill patients, protocols for these advanced services had to be developed on the fly.

EVD Clinical Manifestations—Lessons Learned in Resource-Rich Settings

Following infection by contact with infected bodily fluid, there is an incubation period of 2–21 days prior to the onset of EVD symptoms, which most commonly begin with profound fatigue, headache, poor appetite (anorexia), fevers, muscle and joint pains, and rash.[6] This initial prodromal phase of illness is followed by a gastroenteritis/hepatitis phase characterized by progressive high spiking fevers, nausea with occasional vomiting, and voluminous watery diarrhea (as much as 10–12 L/day). Complications of this brisk diarrhea can include severe electrolyte disturbances and dehydration. Furthermore, there is evidence of liver inflammation (hepatitis) and muscle injury.[7] In the absence of advanced life support measures or inadequate access to basic oral or intravenous rehydration solutions in resource-poor settings, it is during this gastroenteritis/hepatitis phase of illness that most fatalities from EVD occur as a result of complications from diarrhea and dehydration, leading to organ failure and death.[8]

While taking care of a patient with EVD can never be taken lightly or for granted, as biocontainment isolation units in resource-rich settings prepared to possibly care for EVD evacuees, it was felt that mortality rates should be much lower than in West Africa. Specifically, in these settings, ready access to oral and intravenous rehydration options, laboratory support, and electrolyte replacement options would, in theory, minimize the risk of death during this diarrheal phase, allowing for a patient's native immune system to develop a response and clear the infection. Early experience treating EVD in resource-rich settings followed such a pattern, with the first two cases cared for at Emory demonstrating moderate symptoms over these early phases followed by steady decline in viral load and recovery to hospital discharge.[9] Shortly after Emory's initial experience, a UK national contracted EVD in Sierra Leone and was evacuated to London; his course of disease demonstrated a similar pattern to the Emory experience.[10]

While these early experiences demonstrated that supportive care was an effective treatment plan for EVD, concern remained given that these early cases experienced only moderate viral loads[11] as initial and peak viral loads are known to correlate with mortality.[12] Thus, it was acknowledged that the spectrum of clinical effects (phenotype), especially in severe EVD, remained unclear. However, beginning with a third case treated at EUH in September 2014, it became evident that EVD may manifest in a more severe form, leading to multi-organ failure requiring advanced life support, including acute hemodialysis and mechanical ventilation.[13]

This patient at EUH had high viral loads at diagnosis, which progressively increased to markedly high levels over the first 10 days of illness.

The course of disease in this case was characterized, as usual, by high fevers, voluminous diarrhea, acute hepatitis, and poor appetite over the first week. However, beginning approximately on day 8 of illness, the patient's mental status deteriorated, with progressive confusion and encephalopathy. He also developed worsening oxygen levels (hypoxia), respiratory distress, and kidney failure. As a result, on day 9 of illness, with development of progressive respiratory failure, advanced life support was required to prevent his death.[14] Thus, this patient became the first EVD patient in the world known to have been managed with invasive mechanical ventilation and renal replacement therapy (i.e., continuous hemodialysis).[15] Over the next 12 months, approximately 30 total EVD patients have been managed to date in the resource-rich settings of North America and Europe, several of whom became critically ill with severe EVD requiring advanced life support.[16]

Clinical Manifestations of Severe EVD

With the above experiences in resource-rich settings, it has become clear that patients with EVD presenting with high viral loads and high peak viral loads have experienced a common pattern of multi-organ failure. While patients with mild to moderate EVD begin to experience resolution of fever, gastrointestinal, and other symptoms around days 8–10 of illness, patients with severe EVD and high viral loads develop progression of symptoms during days 8–12 of illness, characterized by the development of respiratory distress, pulmonary edema, decreasing urine output, acute kidney failure, and worsening mental status (i.e., encephalopathy).[17] Specifically, respiratory distress and hypoxia have led to respiratory failure, requiring both noninvasive ventilation support and invasive mechanical ventilation. Acute kidney failure has necessitated the use of renal replacement therapy in several reported[18] and unreported cases (personal communication, T. Uyeki, US Centers for Disease Control and Prevention).

By enabling multiple critically ill patients with severe EVD to survive, recover, and ultimately be discharged from the hospital, advanced life support for critical illness has contributed to a decrease in mortality from severe EVD in resource-rich settings (i.e., the United States and Europe) to as low as approximately 20 percent to date. However, despite advanced care options in the United States and Europe, severe EVD remains a potentially fatal disease, with multiple patients experiencing complications, including secondary bacterial infections, abdominal insults, fatal cardiac arrhythmias, and/or death.[19] Unfortunately, given the limitations of care that still persist in biocontainment isolation (i.e., incomplete access to advanced imaging), the terminal events leading to death in fatal cases in the United States and Europe remain unclear.[20]

Management of EVD in Biocontainment Isolation

Biocontainment isolation for life-threatening communicable infectious diseases like EVD is used primarily as a means to isolate the patients from the general population and, more specifically, the greater hospital population (patients and HCWs) in an effort to limit the risk of disease transmission. However, it must be noted that managing a complex disease such as EVD in biocontainment isolation has proven a unique challenge for health care providers used to the comforts of contemporary acute care in modern tertiary hospital settings. All aspects of care are impacted by biocontainment isolation and personal protective equipment (PPE). Physical exams with stethoscopes and other techniques are markedly hampered by PPE, and patients are physically isolated in rooms with immediate access only to a nurse rather than the whole team of HCWs, as is standard in modern advanced health care settings, especially in intensive care units. When caring for a patient in strict biocontainment isolation, safety is of paramount importance and involves attention to patient safety, HCW safety, and population safety.[21]

Patient Safety

Strict biocontainment isolation introduces risk for the patient. Whereas in a typical hospital setting, HCWs are usually readily available to assist a critically ill patient during an acute life-threatening event, in strict biocontainment isolation, there are a limited number of HCWs trained to provide care, and PPE and other barriers slow ease of access to the patient during an emergency situation. For example, if the patient has sudden breathing difficulty, bleeding, or other acute issues, it will take at least 10–15 minutes for additional HCWs to properly and safely don PPE in order to enter the isolation environment.

At the EUH biocontainment facility, a nurse was present inside the isolation room at all times, in full PPE, to care for the patient. Given the diversity of patient clinical needs, the potential need for advanced life support, and the isolation of the nurse from immediate support as discussed above, EUH only utilized intensive care unit nurse specialists with broad nursing expertise and experience to function in this role.

As the complexity of patients' needs increased to include advanced life support, protocols and systems were put in place to help the nurse in the case of an emergency. In modern intensive care units, should an emergency occur—such as failure of mechanical ventilator, unplanned extubation (removal of breathing tube), cardiac arrest, bleeding, or complications from hemodialysis, and so on—help and support for the nurse is immediately available. However, in our biocontainment facility, the nurse would be addressing these sudden events without physical assistance for at least 10–15 minutes while other staff members donned PPE. As such, the nurse needed necessary equipment, training, and support to address these issues as soon as possible in order to maximize patient safety.

HCW Safety

EBOV is transmitted to unprotected HCWs and other caregivers via contact with bodily fluids that contain viable virus (i.e., blood, sweat, gastric contents, stool/diarrhea, urine, semen, etc.). As a result, aside from isolating patients, all HCWs must use extensive PPE to protect themselves from exposure and minimize risk of transfer of the viral particles outside of the isolation environment. While PPE decreases HCW exposure and risk, it does not eliminate risk and can in fact introduce risk of transmission if there are failures of PPE equipment or the donning/doffing procedure.[22] Given that every intervention/interaction with the patient has risk of disease transmission to HCWs, careful planning must be undertaken prior to all routine and, especially, complex interactions.

Maximizing HCW safety must go beyond proper PPE. At EUH, like other institutions, a constant buddy system was used to support all HCWs in PPE in the isolation room by providing easy communication and support in the isolation room. All donning and doffing of PPE is directed step by step and supervised by the buddy. HCW fatigue promotes errors, and wearing PPE causes fatigue quickly; thus, nurses were rotated out of the isolation room every 3–4 hours. Attempts were made to minimize risks of exposure to infected body fluids or possible needle sticks: central venous line for needleless blood draws inserted on admission, batching blood and sample collections, bowel management system to contain diarrhea, and frequent cleaning of environmental surfaces in the isolation room by HCWs. Furthermore, frequent PPE donning/doffing refresher training was provided for less frequent users (e.g., physicians, technicians, etc.). All unnecessary staff entry to isolation room was avoided; one or two physicians would examine the patient daily, and consultants were not admitted to the isolation room unless a necessary procedure or subspecialty-specific intervention was required.

Finally, in resource-rich settings, HCWs and administrations must redefine "success" when treating EVD. Rather than the norm, in which HCWs provide care to acutely ill patients with little regard for their own safety, HCW safety (i.e., no secondary HCW infections) must be included as a barometer of "successful" treatment of EVD or high-risk, highly contagious illnesses like EVD. In other words, rather than a sole focus on patient outcome as is the usual practice in resource-rich settings, successful treatment of EVD should be defined as no secondary transmission while striving for the best possible patient outcome.

Finally, while ethicists correctly argue that HCWs have an ethical duty to treat patients with EVD and other communicable diseases,[23] this does not obviate the necessity to protect HCWs from infection to the fullest extent possible. In West Africa, deaths of HCWs from EVD have devastated an already unacceptably small core of HCWs and will have long-term ramifications on a fragile health care system,[24] with a total of 880 confirmed HCW infections and 512 HCW deaths during the current outbreak.[25]

Population and Community Safety

The final aspect of safety that must be considered is the hospital and population safety at large. EVD-infected patients must be isolated to minimize the risk to the general hospital and the surrounding community. At EUH and other resource-rich settings, this is accomplished by biocontainment isolation, in which patients are quarantined until infection has resolved and the virus has cleared from blood. Biocontainment isolation also necessitates a plan to manage highly infectious human and biomedical waste products. At EUH, local government and health department regulations governed methods for disposal of medical waste and bodily fluids. All medical equipment used on any given patient remained sequestered in the isolation room until terminal decontamination after patient discharge.

Furthermore, to limit risk to the rest of the hospital at EUH, all labs were processed in the biocontainment facility by specially trained lab technicians using point-of-care technology.[26] The isolated EVD patients did not leave the isolation environment for advanced imaging or tests (i.e., no CT scans, MRIs, etc.). Staff underwent rigorous twice-daily temperature monitoring for 21 days after last known EVD contact.

EVD Treatment Options

The only proven effective therapy for EVD remains advanced supportive care. However, almost all patients managed in resource-rich settings have received some combination of experimental therapies in an uncontrolled fashion administered outside rigorous clinical trials in a desperate search for possible new treatment strategies. Bishop recently published a summary of experimental therapies, which have included: 1) humanized monoclonal antibodies (ZMapp); 2) convalescent human plasma (i.e., plasma from EVD survivors to share EVD-specific antibodies); 3) small interfering RNA (TKM-100802); 4) antiviral agents (e.g., brincidofovir, favipiravir, and others).[27] Furthermore, Büttner et al. describe direct virus elimination from blood with a blood-purification technique called lectin affinity plasmapharesis.[28] The patients managed at EUH received ZMapp, TKM-100802, and/or convalescent plasma transfusions.[29] This uncontrolled use of multiple experimental therapies outside of rigorous clinical trials in the early care of EVD in the United States and Europe will make it very difficult to ascertain if any specific therapy was effective. There are now several randomized clinical trials attempting to scientifically evaluate these experimental therapies, including favipiravir (clinicaltrials.gov identifier NCT02329054), ZMapp (clinicaltrials.gov identifier NCT02363322), and convalescent plasma (clinicaltrials.gov identifier NCT02333578). However, as the current outbreak is thankfully waning, the number of patients eligible to enroll in these trials in the United States and Europe will be very limited.

Conclusion

EVD remains a complex, life-threatening illness. The only proven therapy remains advanced supportive care and life support. While biocontainment isolation does introduce new challenges in the care of critically ill patients, experiences around the world with EVD since 2014 have demonstrated that advanced life support can and should be provided safely in biocontainment isolation. While the tragedy of the current 2013–2016 EVD outbreak cannot be overstated, with over 11,000 deaths around the world, the dangers posed by EVD have yielded an invaluable opportunity for global pandemic preparedness to be tested and more robust systems developed. Given the risks of epidemic/pandemic potential posed by serious emerging infections made easier by the speed of global travel in the modern era, it would be disappointing if the lessons learned in the management of EVD around the world in this outbreak do not provide a model for governments, public health, hospitals, and clinicians to develop more robust global infrastructures to better respond in the future.

Notes

1. Mandell, Gerald L., John E. Bennett, and Raphael Dolin, eds. *Mandell, Douglas, and Bennett's Principles and Practice of Infectious Diseases*, 7th ed., vol. 2 (Philadelphia: Churchill Livingstone/Elsevier, 2010).

2. World Health Organization, "Ebola Response Roadmap Situation Report," accessed December 2, 2014, http://www.who.int/csr/disease/ebola/situation-reports/.

3. P. W. Smith, A. O. Anderson, G. W. Christopher, T. J. Cieslak, G. J. Devreede, G. A. Fosdick, et al. "Designing a Biocontainment Unit to Care for Patients with Serious Communicable Diseases: A Consensus Statement," *Biosecurity and Bioterrorism* 4, no. 4 (2006): 351–65, doi: 10.1089/bsp.2006.4.351.

4. Ibid.

5. M. A. Bwaka, M. J. Bonnet, P. Calain, R. Colebunders, A. De Roo, Y. Guimard, et al., "Ebola Hemorrhagic Fever in Kikwit, Democratic Republic of the Congo: Clinical Observations in 103 Patients," *Journal of Infectious Diseases* 179, suppl. 1 (1999): S1–7, doi: 10.1086/514308; C. J. Peters and J. W. LeDuc, "An Introduction to Ebola: The Virus and the Disease," *Journal of Infectious Diseases* 179, suppl. 1 (1999): ix–xvi, doi: 10.1086/514322; H. Feldmann and T. W. Geisbert, "Ebola Haemorrhagic Fever," *The Lancet* 377, no. 9768 (2011): 849–62, doi: 10.1016/S0140-6736(10)60667-8; M. G. Dixon and I. J. Schafer, "Ebola Viral Disease Outbreak—West Africa, 2014," *Morbidity and Mortality Weekly Report* 63, no. 25 (2014): 548–51, doi: mm6325a4; Mandell, Bennett, and Dolin, *Principles and Practice of Infectious Diseases*.

6. Bwaka et al., "Ebola Hemorrhagic Fever in Kikwit, Democratic Republic of the Congo: Clinical Observations in 103 Patients"; Feldmann and Geisbert, "Ebola Haemorrhagic Fever"; R. Ansumana, K. H. Jacobsen, M. Idris, H. Bangura,

M. Boie-Jalloh, J. M. Lamin, et al., "Ebola in Freetown Area, Sierra Leone—A Case Study of 581 Patients," *The New England Journal of Medicine* 372, no. 6 (2015): 587–8, doi: 10.1056/NEJMc1413685.

7. V. Sueblinvong, D. W. Johnson, G. L. Weinstein, M. J. Connor Jr., I. Crozier, A. M. Liddell, et al., "Critical Care for Multiple Organ Failure Secondary to Ebola Virus Disease in the United States," *Critical Care Medicine* 43, no. 10 (2015): 2066–75, doi: 10.1097/CCM.0000000000001197.

8. Feldmann and Geisbert, "Ebola Haemorrhagic Fever."

9. G. M. Lyon, A. K. Mehta, J. B. Varkey, K. Brantly, L. Plyler, A. K. McElroy, et al., "Clinical Care of Two Patients with Ebola Virus Disease in the United States," *The New England Journal of Medicine* 371, no. 25 (2014): 2402–9, doi: 10.1056/NEJMoa1409838.

10. W. Pooley, "Ebola: Perspectives from a Nurse and Patient," *The American Journal of Tropical Medicine and Hygiene* 92, no. 2 (2015): 223–4, doi: 10.4269/ajtmh.14-0762.

11. Lyon et al., "Clinical Care of Two Patients with Ebola Virus Disease in the United States."

12. J. S. Towner, P. E. Rollin, D. G. Bausch, A. Sanchez, S. M. Crary, M. Vincent, et al., "Rapid Diagnosis of Ebola Hemorrhagic Fever by Reverse Transcription-PCR in an Outbreak Setting and Assessment of Patient Viral Load as a Predictor Of Outcome," *Journal of Virology* 78, no, 8 (2004): 4330–41.

13. M. J. Connor Jr., C. Kraft, A. K. Mehta, J. B. Varkey, G. M. Lyon, I. Crozier, et al., "Successful Delivery of RRT in Ebola Virus Disease," *Journal of the American Society of Nephrology* 26, no. 1 (2015): 31–7, doi: ASN.2014111057; C. S. Kraft, A. L. Hewlett, S. Koepsell, A. M. Winkler, C. J. Kratochvil, L. Larson, et al., "The Use of TKM-100802 and Convalescent Plasma in 2 Patients With Ebola Virus Disease in the United States," *Clinical Infectious Diseases* 61, no. 4 (2015): 496–502, doi: 10.1093/cid/civ334.

14. Kraft, "The Use of TKM-100802 and Convalescent Plasma in 2 Patients With Ebola Virus Disease in the United States."

15. Connor et al., "Successful Delivery of RRT in Ebola Virus Disease"; Kraft et al., "The Use of TKM-100802 and Convalescent Plasma in 2 Patients With Ebola Virus Disease in the United States."

16. B. Kreuels, D. Wichmann, P. Emmerich, J. Schmidt-Chanasit, G. de Heer, S. Kluge, et al. "A Case of Severe Ebola Virus Infection Complicated by Gram-Negative Septicemia," *The New England Journal of Medicine* 371, no. 25 (2014): 2394–401, doi: 10.1056/NEJMoa1411677; T. Wolf, G. Kann, S. Becker, C. Stephan, H. R. Brodt, P. de Leuw, et al., "Severe Ebola Virus Disease with Vascular Leakage and Multiorgan Failure: Treatment of a Patient in Intensive Care," *The Lancet* 385, no. 9976 (2014):

1428–35, doi: 10.1016/S0140-6736(14)62384-9; A. M. Liddell, R. T. Davey Jr., A. K. Mehta, J. B. Varkey, C. S. Kraft, G. K. Tseggay, et al., "Characteristics and Clinical Management of a Cluster of 3 Patients With Ebola Virus Disease, Including the First Domestically Acquired Cases in the United States," *Annals of Internal Medicine* 162, no. 2 (2015): 81–90, doi: 10.7326/M15-0530; K. Yacisin, S. Balter, A. Fine, D. Weiss, J. Ackelsberg, D. Prezant, et al., "Ebola Virus Disease in a Humanitarian Aid Worker—New York City, October 2014," *Morbidity and Mortality Weekly Report* 64, no. 12 (2015): 321–3; J. M. Parra, O. J. Salmeron, and M. Velasco, "The First Case of Ebola Virus Disease Acquired outside Africa," *The New England Journal of Medicine* 371, no. 25 (2014): 2439–40, doi: 10.1056/NEJMc1412662; Sueblinvong et al., "Critical Care for Multiple Organ Failure Secondary to Ebola Virus Disease in the United States."

17. Connor et al., "Successful Delivery of RRT in Ebola Virus Disease"; Kraft et al., "The Use of TKM-100802 and Convalescent Plasma in 2 Patients With Ebola Virus Disease in the United States"; Liddell et al., "Characteristics and Clinical Management of a Cluster of 3 Patients With Ebola Virus Disease, Including the First Domestically Acquired Cases in the United States"; Wolf et al., "Severe Ebola Virus Disease with Vascular Leakage and Multiorgan Failure: Treatment of a Patient in Intensive Care"; Kreuels et al., "A Case of Severe Ebola Virus Infection Complicated by Gram-Negative Septicemia"; Sueblinvong et al., "Critical Care for Multiple Organ Failure Secondary to Ebola Virus Disease in the United States."

18. Connor et al., "Successful Delivery of RRT in Ebola Virus Disease"; Kraft et al., "The Use of TKM-100802 and Convalescent Plasma in 2 Patients With Ebola Virus Disease in the United States"; Liddell et al., "Characteristics and Clinical Management of a Cluster of 3 Patients With Ebola Virus Disease, Including the First Domestically Acquired Cases in the United States"; Sueblinvong et al., "Critical Care for Multiple Organ Failure Secondary to Ebola Virus Disease in the United States"; S. Büttner, B. Koch, O. Dolnik, M. Eickmann, T. Freiwald, S. Rudolf, et al., "Extracorporeal Virus Elimination for the Treatment of Severe Ebola Virus Disease—First Experience with Lectin Affinity Plasmapheresis," *Blood Purification* 38, no. 3–4 (2014): 286–91, doi: 10.1159/000375229.

19. Liddell et al., "Characteristics and Clinical Management of a Cluster of 3 Patients With Ebola Virus Disease, Including the First Domestically Acquired Cases in the United States"; Sueblinvong et al., "Critical Care for Multiple Organ Failure Secondary to Ebola Virus Disease in the United States"; Wolf et al., "Severe Ebola Virus Disease with Vascular Leakage and Multiorgan Failure: Treatment of a Patient in Intensive Care"; Kreuels et al., "A Case of Severe Ebola Virus Infection Complicated by Gram-Negative Septicemia."

20. Sueblinvong et al., "Critical Care for Multiple Organ Failure Secondary to Ebola Virus Disease in the United States."

21. Connor et al., "Successful Delivery of RRT in Ebola Virus Disease."

22. R. A. Fowler, T. Fletcher, W. A. Fischer 2nd, F. Lamontagne, S. Jacob, D. Brett-Major, et al., "Caring for Critically Ill Patients with Ebola Virus Disease. Perspectives from West Africa," *American Journal of Respiratory and Critical Care Medicine* 190, no. 7 (2014): 733–7, doi: 10.1164/rccm.201408-1514CP.

23. N. G. Evans, "Balancing the Duty to Treat Patients with Ebola Virus Disease with the Risks to Dialysis Personnel," *Clinical Journal of the American Society of Nephrology*, August 2015, epub ahead of print, doi: 10.2215/CJN.03730415.

24. Evans, D. K., M. Goldstein, and A. Popova, "Health Care Worker Mortality and the Legacy of the Ebola Epidemic," *The Lancet Global Health* 3, no. 8 (2015): e439–40, doi: 10.1016/S2214-109X(15)00065-0.

25. World Health Organization, "Ebola response roadmap situation report."

26. C. E. Hill, E. M. Burd, C. S. Kraft, E. L. Ryan, A. Duncan, A. M. Winkler, et al., "Laboratory Test Support for Ebola Patients within a High-Containment Facility," *Laboratory Med* 45, no. 3 (2014): e109–11, doi: 10.1309/LMTMW3VVN20HIFS.

27. B. M. Bishop, "Potential and Emerging Treatment Options for Ebola Virus Disease," *Annals of Pharmacotherapy* 49, no. 2 (2015): 196–206, doi: 10.1177/1060028014561227.

28. Büttner et al., "Extracorporeal Virus Elimination for the Treatment of Severe Ebola Virus Disease—First Experience with Lectin Affinity Plasmapheresis."

29. Lyon et al., "Clinical care of two patients with Ebola virus disease in the United States"; Kraft et al., "The Use of TKM-100802 and Convalescent Plasma in 2 Patients With Ebola Virus Disease in the United States."

II The Spread of the 2013–2016 Ebola Virus Disease Outbreak

4 Modeling the Ebola Epidemic: Challenges and Lessons for the Future

Christian L. Althaus

Background

Analyzing infectious disease dynamics by means of mathematics has a long history, going back as far as the late sixteenth and early seventeenth century when plague epidemics raged through Europe.[1] Modern infectious disease epidemiology became established in the second half of the twentieth century[2] and has proven to play a key role in understanding the spread of infectious diseases. At the center of this discipline lies the formulation of mathematical models that describe the contact between susceptible and infectious individuals in order to study the dynamics of transmission over time. Arguably the most important quantity in infectious disease epidemiology is the basic reproduction number, R_0.[3,4,5] This quantity is defined as the average number of new infections caused by a typical infected individual in a population that is completely susceptible (figure 4.1). Knowledge of this quantity provides crucial information about the potential impact of control interventions. As an example, newest estimates of R_0 for measles lie around 30, meaning that one person infected with measles will on average transmit the infection to 30 other people in a population that is unvaccinated and has never before been exposed to the measles virus.[6,7] The high value of R_0 for measles explains the high vaccination rate (~95%) that is required to eliminate measles in a population.[7] On the other hand, seasonal influenza virus has an R_0 around 2, meaning that even small levels of effective vaccination, paired with hygiene measures, can limit transmission to a certain extent.[8]

Until the Ebola virus disease (EVD) outbreak in West Africa, relatively little was known about the transmission dynamics of EVD. In 2004, Chowell et al.[9] published the first estimates of the basic reproduction number for

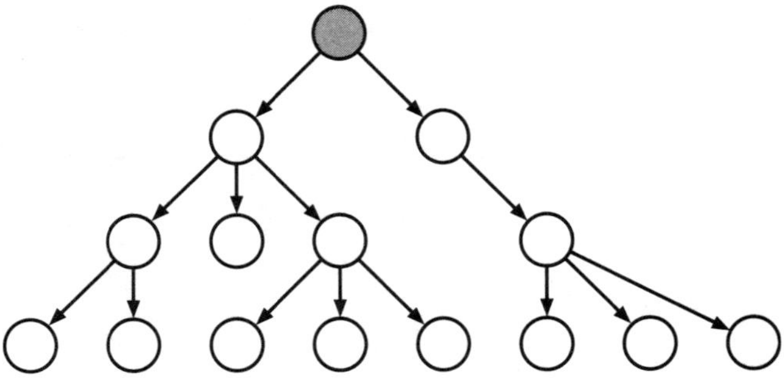

Figure 4.1
Schematic illustration of the basic reproduction number, R_0. When the population is completely susceptible and $R_0 = 2$, the first infectious case (gray circle) generates on average two secondary cases, each of which in turn generates two additional cases on average, and so forth.

two previous EVD outbreaks in the Democratic Republic of Congo ($R_0 = 1.8$) and Uganda ($R_0 = 1.3$). These relatively low estimates of R_0 indicated that EVD is not highly transmissible unless individuals are in direct contact with body fluids of an infected person and that control interventions such as case isolation, quarantine, and contact tracing have the potential to reduce transmission significantly. Apart from a notable second study published by Legrand et al.,[10] analyzing the transmission dynamics of EVD received little notice in the scientific community. However, this changed dramatically with the emergence of EVD in West Africa, a region that had never reported an EVD outbreak before 2013.

First Months of the Outbreak

It is now believed that the first case of the EVD outbreak in West Africa was a two-year-old child from the prefecture of Guéckédou in Guinea.[11] The child likely contracted the virus from an animal reservoir and died on 6 December 2013, infecting other family members along the way. The outbreak remained unnoticed until March 2014, when teams of the health ministry and Médecins sans Frontières (MSF) started an investigation. One month later, the *New England Journal of Medicine* published the first study describing the emergence of EVD in Guinea.[11] The outbreak received limited attention in the following months before the rapid increase in the number of infected cases caused the World Health Organization (WHO) to call the outbreak a public health emergency of international concern (PHEIC) on August 8, 2014.[12]

The initial lack of studies investigating the outbreak dynamics was rather atypical for an outbreak of an emergent infectious disease. Other outbreaks, such as severe acute respiratory syndrome coronavirus (SARS-CoV) in 2003, H1N1 pandemic influenza in 2009, and Middle East respiratory syndrome coronavirus (MERS-CoV) in 2012 saw the rapid publication of early outbreak analyses with descriptions of the transmission dynamics and estimates of R_0.[13,14,15,16] These studies helped assess epidemic potential and impact of control interventions in real time. In contrast, there was still inadequate understanding of the outbreak dynamics of EVD in the three affected countries by summer 2014. This was all the more surprising as the reported cumulative number of clinical cases and deaths climbed to 1,603 and 887 respectively by August 1, 2014,[17] including four cases from an additional outbreak caused by an infected air traveler who exported the disease to Nigeria via the international airport in Lagos.[18,19]

Early Studies on Transmission Dynamics

At the beginning of August 2014, there was no study yet describing the transmission dynamics and basic reproduction number for the West African EVD outbreak. However, several researchers started to collect data from various websites from the WHO and local ministries of health that had published case data, and compiled data files that allowed them to analyze the different epidemic curves in the affected countries. Althaus[17] constructed a mathematical model—similar in fashion to the first model developed by Chowell et al.[9]—with different compartments that describe the transmission of EVD from infected to susceptible individuals and how infected individuals recover from the disease or die. Fitting this model to the data resulted in the first estimates of the basic reproduction number of EVD for each country. Furthermore, the model provided insights into whether control interventions had already led to a reduction in transmission. What the study showed was reassuring as well as frightening. The values of R_0 in Guinea, Sierra Leone, and Liberia ranged between 1.5 and 2.5.[17] They were very similar to the estimates from previous outbreaks,[9,10] indicating that the transmissibility of EVD had not changed and that implementing the control interventions that had been used previously would limit further spread. Indeed, the model results showed that a certain level of control had been achieved in Guinea and Sierra Leone during May and July 2014. In stark contrast, the results also showed that the epidemic was completely out of control in Liberia, where the number of infected cases and deaths due to EVD continued to grow exponentially and was doubling every two weeks (figure 4.2). The study was initially published on arXiv, an open-access repository for electronic preprints, and later appeared in *PLOS Currents: Outbreaks*, a specialized scientific journal that undertakes rapid peer review and was designed for such emergency situations, on September 2, 2014.[17] The study's findings were corroborated by a number of other modeling studies that were published in the days and weeks that followed.[20,21,22,23]

The WHO Ebola Response Team published their long-awaited study describing the outbreak dynamics in great detail in the second half of September 2014.[24] The infectious disease epidemiologists from the WHO

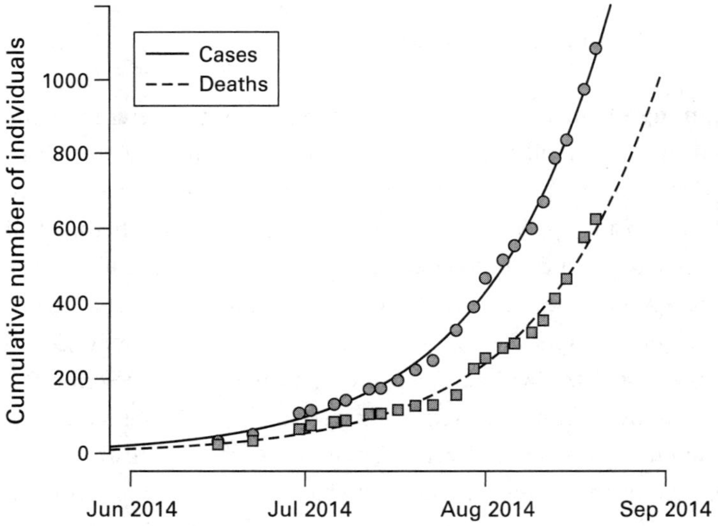

Figure 4.2
Dynamics of Ebola virus disease (EVD) outbreak in Liberia up to the end of August 2014. Reported data of the cumulative numbers of infected cases and deaths are shown as circles and squares, respectively. The lines represent the fit of the mathematical model to the data. Figure adapted from Althaus.[17]

and their collaborators had access to clinical data that included the dates of symptom onset and hospitalization, and the time at which the patients had contact with other persons who had EVD. This allowed the researchers to study infection characteristics such as the incubation period, which is the time between infection and onset of symptoms. Knowing the length of this period was important for assessing the duration during which case contacts needed to be followed up. Furthermore, the study provided a detailed picture of the generation time (time between infection in an index case and infection in a patient infected by said index case), which allowed for more accurate estimates of R_0. Overall, the WHO study came to the conclusion that the infection characteristics of EVD were similar to what had been observed in smaller outbreaks during the past decades. Nevertheless, a pessimistic outlook on the course of the outbreak remained. Assuming no change in control measures that would lead to a decrease in the reproduction number, the authors predicted that the cumulative number of cases in all three countries could exceed 20,000 by the beginning of November 2014.[24] Another study used a similar method but extrapolated the number of cases until the end of 2014 and found that 77,181 to 277,124 cases would be expected by then.[22] Around the same time, the US Centers for Disease Control and Prevention published a report with the most catastrophic scenario. They argued that the true number of EVD cases could be 2.5 times higher than reported and calculated that Sierra Leone and Liberia could reach 1.4 million cases by January 20, 2015, if this correction factor for underreporting was taken into account.[25]

While such long-term forecasts are error-prone, all these studies clearly highlighted that the epidemic was completely rampant and growing exponentially in certain areas. With such large numbers of infected cases to be expected, would traditional control measures such as case isolation, quarantine, and contact tracing still be feasible? Or was there a critical point beyond which it would prove almost impossible to manage the outbreak? Several studies also approached these questions by incorporating various control interventions into their mathematical models. For example, it is possible to simulate isolation of infected patients by moving infected individuals into another compartment where they could not transmit the disease further. These real-time studies provided important insights into the proportion of patients that needed to be hospitalized,[26] the required number of hospital beds,[27] and the benefits and risks of introducing community care centers to isolate suspected cases.[28]

Another factor of uncertainty was the impact of traditional funeral practices—which can involve washing, touching, or kissing of the body—on EVD transmission. The journal *Science* published a controversial modeling study suggesting that funeral transmission alone could sustain the epidemic in Liberia.[29] However, it is exceedingly difficult to quantify the separate contribution of community, hospital, and funeral transmission,[30] and the result of this particular study was based on various model assumptions about the risk of acquiring the infection at a funeral of a person who died of EVD. Other studies—of which some were based on epidemiological contact tracing—showed that the amount of funeral transmission was minor and contributed around 10% to overall transmission.[24,31,32]

Concomitant with the publication of these modeling studies, the international aid to contain the epidemic in West Africa increased dramatically. The weekly numbers of new EVD cases that were reported started to decline after October 2014. How much of this decline can be attributed to the increase in health care capacities remains a matter of debate. Additional factors, such as behavior change in the population due to increased awareness, could have led to a reduction in transmission and might have supported the effect of the newly introduced control interventions.

Challenges

The website of the WHO Regional Office for Africa began publishing regular updates about the epidemiology and surveillance of the outbreak after March 2014.[33] While this proved useful as scientists around the world could access the data, there were several major problems. First, there was considerable uncertainty around the data, as they were not assembled in a coordinated manner. Second, not all reported cases were laboratory-confirmed, and it was unclear whether this led to over- or underreporting of the actual number of cases. Third, the case numbers were mostly reported as cumulative numbers and at irregular intervals. This, and the fact that cases were sometimes reclassified as non-cases, complicated the calculation of the number of new infections observed every week. Finally, the data were presented as text or in tables in HTML or PDF documents. This made it difficult to automatically download the data using customized software tools.

Caitlin Rivers, who was at the time a graduate student in computational epidemiology at Virginia Tech, aggregated the available data from the WHO outbreak news, situation reports, and the local ministries of health into machine-readable files and made them publicly available on her GitHub repository.[34] This made it much easier for other research groups to quickly access the most recent data to analyze the outbreak dynamics. At the peak of the epidemic, the WHO redesigned their website and began publishing up-to-date situation reports,[35] making it substantially easier to access and analyze the epidemiological data in real time. If these features had been available during spring 2014, researchers would have been able to analyze the epidemic trajectory much earlier. An understanding of the scale of the outbreak early on, and showing that the epidemic was out of control in some areas, might have helped inspire an earlier international response to the outbreak. This missed opportunity was mentioned in a report from the WHO Ebola Interim Assessment Panel published in July 2015, which stated that "data were not aggregated, analysed or shared in a timely manner and in some cases not at all."[36]

Another challenge is the inherent uncertainty in analyzing and interpreting epidemiological data and in making predictions about the future course of an epidemic. Small changes in model assumptions and parameters can lead to wildly different outcomes, in particular for long-term model projections as discussed above. Nevertheless, such models can still be useful to study worst-case scenarios and the type of interventions that would be needed to prevent them from happening. Estimating the probability of rare events also proves difficult, in particular if there is no previous information about such events. For example, several studies assessed the potential for international spread of EVD through air travel.[20,37,38] These studies made use of worldwide airline passenger data and came to the conclusion that the short-term probability of international spread was small but not negligible. Indeed, infected cases that traveled outside West Africa spread EVD to several countries. But to predict exactly which country would be affected proved nearly impossible. These two examples—epidemic forecasting and assessing the potential for international spread—illustrate the potential and limitations of mathematical models.

The ways in which some modeling studies were presented, interpreted, and communicated led to substantial criticism, and their use for public health policy making was sometimes met with resistance. A news piece in the journal *Nature* noted that model forecasts were not in line with the observed trajectory of the epidemic in Liberia and overestimated the number of cases during October 2014.[39] However, the projections cited in the piece were worst-case scenarios, and assumed that containment measures were ineffective and transmission did not change through other means. A group of modelers responded to this criticism and argued that focusing on the failure of models to project the epidemic accurately undervalues their other aims.[40] While the models played a role in informing the international response, they were also important tools for synthesizing and incorporating data from multiple sources to create a summary picture that could help guide decision makers during an epidemic.[41]

Lessons to Learn

Retrospectively, the EVD outbreak in West Africa has taught the scientific community several lessons on how to respond to similar events in the future. On one hand, the outbreak demonstrated how mathematical modeling of infectious diseases could provide crucial information for anticipating transmission dynamics and potential impact of control interventions. On the other hand, it became clear that several factors prevented the full potential of models from being realized during the outbreak. Some guidelines on what could be improved to enhance the use of models in outbreak situations follow:

1. Epidemiological data should be readily accessible during the early phase of an outbreak. This requires a collaborative effort of local authorities and health ministries with international organizations such as the WHO. Rapid data sharing will allow experts in the field of mathematical and computational epidemiology to analyze the outbreak in real time and to provide recommendations for policy makers. The MERS-CoV outbreak in South Korea from May to July 2015 represents a promising example where the epidemic curve of the outbreak was published in real time.[42]
2. Line lists that contain information about infected individuals such as age, sex, date of symptom onset, and infection outcome should be made available in machine-readable file formats, such as comma-separated values. This will facilitate the automated analyses of newly released data sets and prevents errors that could otherwise happen

during data processing. Sharing of such information can pose privacy issues, and standardized protocols need to be established by the respective health agencies and ministries to better protect patients.[43]

3. Alternative data sources that could improve our understanding of infectious disease transmission in a particular geographical area should be considered.[44] For example, maps of human mobility based on mobile phone network data[45] or high-resolution data on human population distributions[46] could help improve the parameterization of infectious disease models.
4. The scientific research community should aim for rapid dissemination of their results and publish them via open-access journals, in addition to the use of digital repositories (e.g., GitHub). While it might be more prestigious to publish early outbreak analyses in leading subscription-based journals, publications in open-access journals often receive more citations, thus providing an incentive for academic researchers.[47] Before publication in peer-reviewed journals, manuscripts could be made available through the use of preprint servers such as arXiv, bioRxiv, or PeerJ Preprints.
5. Mathematical modelers should be upfront about the potential and limitations of their models and results. Modelers should think carefully about what is really known about the transmission of the pathogen and the impact of interventions, as well as highlight the assumptions they made to come to their conclusions. In particular, modelers need to clearly distinguish between results that are inferred from data (data-driven) and results that are based on model assumptions (assumption-driven).
6. The results of modeling studies should be relayed in a balanced way, particularly when communicating with the media. Scientists should do their best to clarify the inherent uncertainties around their results and projections and should make sure there is little room for misinterpretation of their statements.

The last decades have shown an increasing trend in emergent and re-emergent infectious diseases.[48] Climate change, increased population density, and human mobility will likely lead to new infectious disease outbreaks in the years to come. The points mentioned above highlight just a few important aspects, but taking them into consideration will likely result in a better use of mathematical modeling for future outbreaks of emerging and re-emerging infectious diseases. During the 2013–2016 outbreak of EVD, the modeling community was caught by surprise. If we don't learn from the mistakes that we made, we could again face a situation where important insights from modeling studies appear a little too late.

Funding Statement

Christian L. Althaus received funding through an Ambizione grant from the Swiss National Science Foundation (SNSF).

Acknowledgments

I would like to thank my co-workers and collaborators, particularly Sandro Gsteiger and Fabienne Krauer, for contributing to the projects related to the Ebola outbreak in West Africa.

Notes

1. Alfredo Morabia, *A History of Epidemiologic Methods and Concepts* (Basel: Birkhauser Verlag, 2004).

2. Roy M. Anderson and Robert M. May. *Infectious Diseases of Humans: Dynamics and Control* (Oxford: Oxford University Press, 1991).

3. O. Diekmann, J. A. Heesterbeek, and J. A. Metz, "On the Definition and the Computation of the Basic Reproduction Ratio *R*0 in Models for Infectious Diseases in Heterogeneous Populations," *Journal of Mathematical Biology* 28, no. 4 (1990): 365–82.

4. J. A. P. Heesterbeek, "A Brief History of R0 and a Recipe for Its Calculation," *Acta Biotheoretica* 50, no. 3 (2002): 189–204.

5. J. M. Heffernan, R. J. Smith, and L. M. Wahl, "Perspectives on the Basic Reproductive Ratio," *Journal of the Royal Society Interface* 2, no. 4 (2005).

6. Daihai He, Edward L. Ionides, and Aaron A. King, "Plug-and-Play inference for Disease Dynamics: Measles in Large and Small Populations as a Case Study," *Journal of the Royal Society Interface* 7, no. 43 (2010): 271–83.

7. Michiel van Boven, Mirjam Kretzschmar, Jacco Wallinga, Philip D. O'Neill, Ole Wichmann, and Susan Hahné, "Estimation of Measles Vaccine Efficacy and Critical Vaccination Coverage in a Highly Vaccinated Population," *Journal of the Royal Society Interface* 7, no. 52 (2010): 1537–44.

8. Marc Baguelin, Stefan Flasche, Anton Camacho, Nikolaos Demiris, Elizabeth Miller, and W. John Edmunds, "Assessing Optimal Target Populations for Influenza Vaccination Programmes: An Evidence Synthesis and Modelling Study," *PLOS Medicine* 10, no. 10 (2013): e1001527.

9. G. Chowell, N. W. Hengartner, C. Castillo-Chavez, P. W. Fenimore, and J. M. Hyman, "The Basic Reproductive Number of Ebola and the Effects of Public Health Measures: The Cases of Congo and Uganda," *Journal of Theoretical Biology* 229, no. 1 (2004): 119–26.

10. J. Legrand, R. F. Grais, P. Y. Boelle, A. J. Valleron, and A. Flahault, "Understanding the Dynamics of Ebola Epidemics," *Epidemiology and Infection* 135, no. 4 (2007): 610–21.

11. Sylvain Baize, Delphine Pannetier, Lisa Oestereich, Toni Rieger, Lamine Koivogui, N'Faly Magassouba, et al., "Emergence of Zaire Ebola Virus Disease in Guinea," *The New England Journal of Medicine* 371, no. 15 (2014): 1418–25.

12. World Health Organization, "Statement on the 1st Meeting of the IHR Emergency Committee on the 2014 Ebola Outbreak in West Africa," August 8, 2014, http://www.who.int/mediacentre/news/statements/2014/ebola-20140808/en/.

13. Marc Lipsitch, Ted Cohen, Ben Cooper, James M. Robins, Stefan Ma, Lyn James, et al., "Transmission Dynamics and Control of Severe Acute Respiratory Syndrome," *Science* 300, no. 5627 (2003): 1966–70.

14. Steven Riley, Christophe Fraser, Christl A. Donnelly, Azra C. Ghani, Laith J. Abu-Raddad, Anthony J. Hedley, et al., "Transmission Dynamics of the Etiological Agent of SARS in Hong Kong: Impact of Public Health interventions," *Science* 300, no. 5627 (2003): 1961–6.

15. Christophe Fraser, Christl A. Donnelly, Simon Cauchemez, William P. Hanage, Maria D. Van Kerkhove, T. Déirdre Hollingsworth, et al., "Pandemic Potential of a Strain of Influenza A (H1N1): Early Findings," *Science* 324, no. 5934 (2009): 1557–61.

16. Romulus Breban, Julien Riou, and Arnaud Fontanet, "Interhuman Transmissibility of Middle East Respiratory Syndrome Coronavirus: Estimation of Pandemic Risk," *The Lancet* 382, no. 9893 (2013): 694–9.

17. Christian L. Althaus, "Estimating the Reproduction Number of Ebola Virus (EBOV) during the 2014 Outbreak in West Africa," *PLOS Currents* 6 (2014).

18. Faisal Shuaib, Rajni Gunnala, Emmanuel O. Musa, Frank J. Mahoney, Olukayode Oguntimehin, Patrick M. Nguku, et al., "Ebola Virus Disease Outbreak—Nigeria, July-September 2014," *Morbidity and Mortality Weekly Report* 63, no. 39 (2014): 867–72.

19. C. L. Althaus, N. Low, E.O. Musa, F. Shuaib, and S. Gsteiger, "Ebola Virus Disease Outbreak in Nigeria: Transmission Dynamics and Rapid Control," *Epidemics* 11 (2015): 80–84.

20. Marcelo F. C. Gomes, Ana Pastore y Piontti, Luca Rossi, Dennis Chao, Ira Longini, M. Elizabeth Halloran, et al., "Assessing the International Spreading Risk Associated with the 2014 West African Ebola Outbreak," *PLOS Currents* 6 (2014).

21. David Fisman, Edwin Khoo, and Ashleigh Tuite, "Early Epidemic Dynamics of the West African 2014 Ebola Outbreak: Estimates Derived with a Simple Two-Parameter Model," *PLOS Currents* 6 (2014).

22. H. Nishiura and G. Chowell, "Early Transmission Dynamics of Ebola Virus Disease (EVD), West Africa, March to August 2014," *Euro Surveillance* 19 (2014): 36.

23. S. Towers, O. Patterson-Lomba, and C. Castillo-Chavez, "Temporal Variations in the Effective Reproduction Number of the 2014 West Africa Ebola Outbreak," *PLOS Currents* 6 (2014).

24. WHO Ebola Response Team, "Ebola Virus Disease in West Africa—The First 9 Months of the Epidemic and Forward Projections," *The New England Journal of Medicine* 371, no. 16 (2014): 1481–95.

25. Martin I. Meltzer, Charisma Y. Atkins, Scott Santibanez, Barbara Knust, Brett W. Petersen, Elizabeth D. Ervin, et al., "Estimating the Future Number of Cases in the Ebola Epidemic—Liberia and Sierra Leone, 2014–2015," *MMWR Surveillance Summaries* 63 (September 2014): 1–14.

26. John M. Drake, RajReni B. Kaul, Laura W. Alexander, Suzanne M. O'Regan, Andrew M. Kramer, J. Tomlin Pulliam, et al., "Ebola Cases and Health System Demand in Liberia," *PLoS Biology* 13, no. 1 (2015): e1002056.

27. Anton Camacho, Adam Kucharski, Yvonne Aki-Sawyerr, Mark A. White, Stefan Flasche, Marc Baguelin, et al., "Temporal Changes in Ebola Transmission in Sierra Leone and Implications for Control Requirements: A Real-time Modelling Study," *PLOS Currents* 7 (2015).

28. Adam J. Kucharski, Anton Camacho, Francesco Checchi, Ron Waldman, Rebecca F. Grais, Jean-Clement Cabrol, et al., "Evaluation of the Benefits and Risks of Introducing Ebola Community Care Centers, Sierra Leone," *Emerging Infectious Diseases* 21, no. 3 (2015): 393–9.

29. Abhishek Pandey, Katherine E. Atkins, Jan Medlock, Natasha Wenzel, Jeffrey P. Townsend, James E. Childs, et al., "Strategies for Containing Ebola in West Africa," *Science* 346, no. 6212 (2014): 991–5.

30. Joshua S. Weitz and Jonathan Dushoff, "Modeling Post-death Transmission of Ebola: Challenges for Inference and Opportunities for Control," *Nature Scientific Reports* 5 (2015): 8751.

31. Stefano Merler, Marco Ajelli, Laura Fumanelli, Marcelo F. C. Gomes, Ana Pastore Y. Piontti, Luca Rossi, et al., "Spatiotemporal Spread of the 2014 Outbreak of Ebola Virus Disease in Liberia and the Effectiveness of Non-Pharmaceutical Interventions: A Computational Modelling Analysis," *The Lancet Infectious Diseases* 15, no. 2 (2015): 204–11.

32. Ousmane Faye, Pierre-Yves Boëlle, Emmanuel Heleze, Oumar Faye, Cheikh Loucoubar, N'Faly Magassouba, et al., "Chains of Transmission and Control of Ebola Virus Disease in Conakry, Guinea, in 2014: An Observational Study," *The Lancet Infectious Diseases* 15, no. 3 (2015): 320–6.

33. World Health Organization, "Disease Outbreak News—WHO Regional office for Africa," accessed August 14, 2015, http://www.afro.who.int/en/clusters-a-programmes/dpc/epidemic-a-pandemic-alert-and-response/outbreak-news.html.

34. Caitlin Rivers, "Data for the 2014 Global Ebola Outbreak," GitHub, accessed August 14, 2015, https://github.com/cmrivers/ebola.

35. World Health Organization, "Ebola Data and Statistics," accessed August 14, 2015, http://apps.who.int/gho/data/node.ebola-sitrep.

36. World Health Organization, "Report of the Ebola Interim Assessment Panel," accessed August 14, 2015, http://www.who.int/csr/resources/publications/ebola/ebola-panel-report/en/.

37. Isaac I. Bogoch, Maria I. Creatore, Martin S. Cetron, John S. Brownstein, Nicki Pesik, Jennifer Miniota, et al., "Assessment of the Potential for International Dissemination of Ebola Virus Via Commercial Air Travel During the 2014 West African Outbreak," *The Lancet* 385, no. 9962 (2015): 29–35.

38. C. Poletto, M. F. Gomes, A. Pastore y Piontti, L. Rossi, L. Bioglio, D. L. Chao, et al., "Assessing the Impact of Travel Restrictions on International Spread of the 2014 West African Ebola Epidemic," *Euro Surveillance* 19, no. 42 (2014).

39. Declan Butler, "Models Overestimate Ebola Cases," *Nature* 515, no. 7525 (2014): 18.

40. Caitlin Rivers, "Ebola: Models Do More Than Forecast," *Nature* 515, no. 7528 (2014): 492.

41. Eric T. Lofgren, M. Elizabeth Halloran, Caitlin M. Rivers, John M. Drake, Travis C. Porco, Bryan Lewis, et al., "Opinion: Mathematical Models: A Key Tool for Outbreak Response," *Proceedings of the National Academy of Sciences USA* 111, no. 51 (2014): 18095–6.

42. World Health Organization, "Middle East Respiratory Syndrome Coronavirus (MERS-CoV)," accessed August 14, 2015, http://www.who.int/emergencies/mers-cov/en/.

43. Nathan L. Yozwiak, Stephen F. Schaffner, and Pardis C. Sabeti, "Data Sharing: Make Outbreak Research Open Access," *Nature* 518, no. 7540 (2015): 477.

44. M. Elizabeth Halloran, Alessandro Vespignani, Nita Bharti, Leora R. Feldstein, K. A. Alexander, Matthew Ferrari, et al., "Ebola: Mobility Data," *Science* 346, no. 6208 (2014): 433.

45. Flowminder Foundation, accessed August 14, 2015, http://www.flowminder.org.

46. Worldpop. "Latest Map," accessed August 14, 2015, http://www.worldpop.org.uk.

47. *Nature*. "Nature Communications data shows open access articles have more views and downloads," *Nature*, press release, July 30, 2014, http://www.nature.com/press_releases/ncomms-report.html.

48. David M. Morens, Gregory K. Folkers, and Anthony S. Fauci, "The Challenge of Emerging and Re-emerging Infectious Diseases," *Nature* 430, no. 6996 (2004): 242–9.

5 Outbreak of Ebola Virus Disease in Guinea: Where Ecology Meets Economy

Daniel G. Bausch and Lara Schwarz

Ebola virus is back, this time in West Africa, with over 350 cases and a 69% case fatality ratio at the time of this writing [2014].[1] The culprit is the Zaire ebolavirus species, the most lethal Ebola virus known, with case fatality ratios up to 90%. The epicenter and site of first introduction is the region of Guéckédou in Guinea's remote southeastern forest region, spilling over into various other regions of Guinea as well as to neighboring Liberia and Sierra Leone (figure 5.1). News of this outbreak engenders three basic questions: (1) What in the world is Zaire ebolavirus doing in West Africa, far from its usual haunts in Central Africa? (2) Why Guinea, where no Ebola virus has ever been seen before? (3) Why now? We'll have to wait for the outbreak to conclude and more data analysis to occur to answer these questions in detail, and even then we may never know, but some educated speculation may be illustrative.

The Ebolavirus genus is comprised of five species, Zaire, Sudan, Taï Forest, Bundibugyo, and Reston, each associated with a consistent case fatality and more or less well-identified endemic area (figure 5.2). Zaire ebolavirus had been previously found only in three Central African countries—the Democratic Republic of the Congo, Republic of the Congo, and Gabon. Thus, the logical assumption when Ebola virus turned up in Guinea was that this would be the Taï Forest species previously noted in Guinea's neighbor, Côte d'Ivoire.

How did Zaire ebolavirus get all the way over to West Africa? The two possibilities appear to be that the virus has always been present in the region, but we just never noticed, or that it was recently introduced. The initial report and phylogenetic analyses on the Guinea outbreak suggested that the Zaire ebolavirus found in Guinea is a distinct strain from that noted in Central Africa,[1] thus suggesting that the virus may not be a

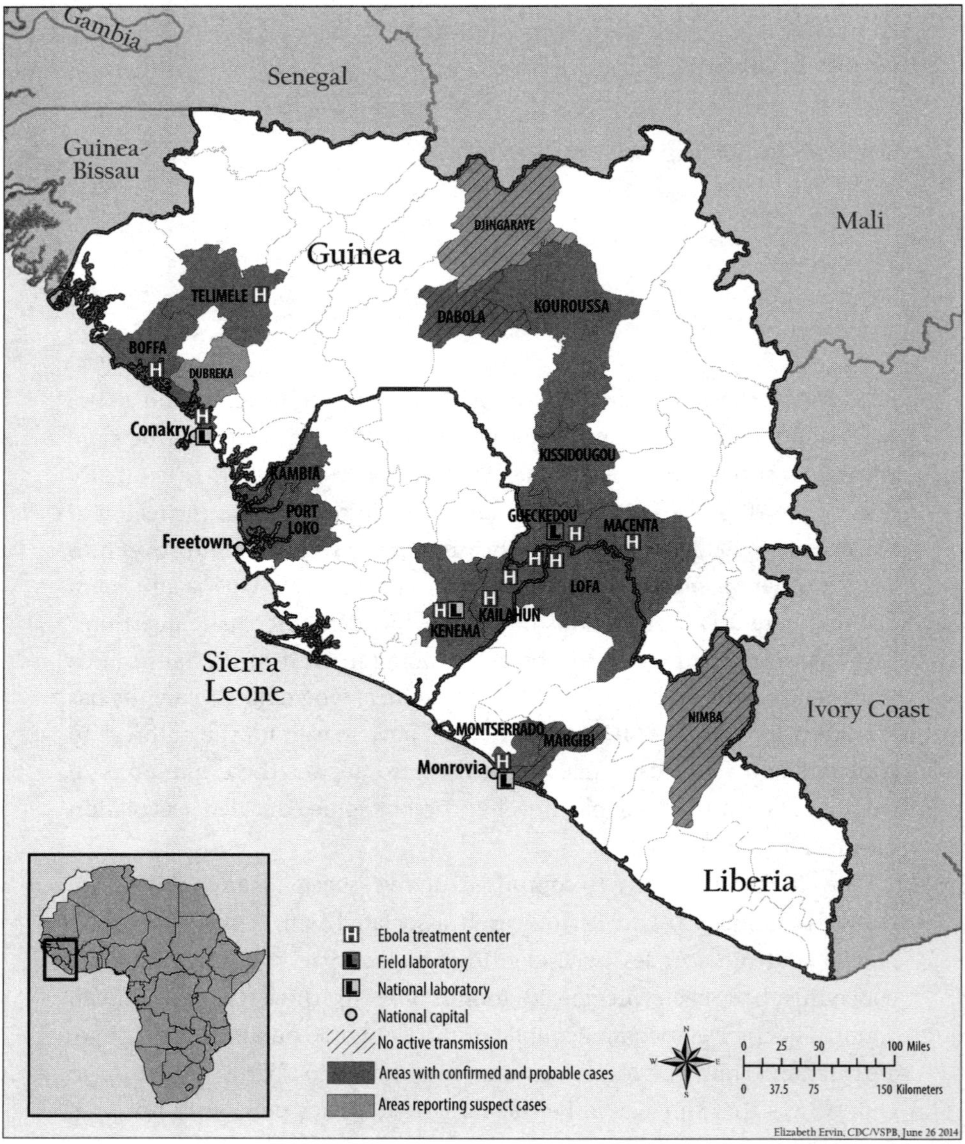

Figure 5.1
Map of the three countries (Guinea, Liberia, and Sierra Leone) involved in the 2013–2014 outbreak of Ebola virus disease as of June 20, 2014. The putative first virus introduction and epicenter are in the vicinity of the town of Guéckédou in the Guinea Forest Region. (Source: CDC; http://www.cdc.gov/vhf/ebola/resources/distribution-map-guinea-outbreak.html.)

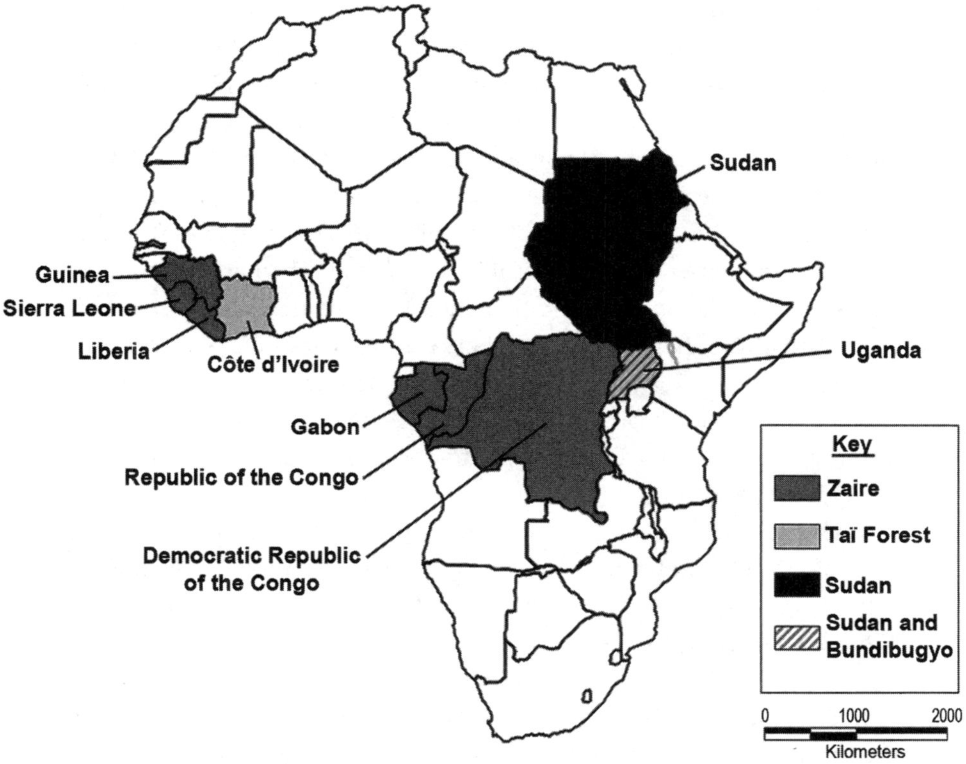

Figure 5.2
African countries where endemic transmission of Ebola virus has been noted.

newcomer to the region. However, subsequent reworking and interpretations of the limited genetic data have cast some doubt on this conclusion.[2] If Zaire ebolavirus had been circulating for some time in Guinea, one might expect greater sequence variation than the 97% homogeneity noted relative to that isolated from Central Africa.[1]

Phylogenetic arguments aside, if Ebola virus was present in Guinea, wouldn't we have seen cases before? Not necessarily. Many pathogens may be maintained in animals with which humans normally have little contact, thus providing limited opportunity for infection. Furthermore, the proportion of infected animals may often be very low, so even frequent contact may not result in pathogen transmission. Even if human Ebola virus infection has occurred, it may not be recognized; contrary to popular conception, the clinical presentation of viral hemorrhagic fever is often very nonspecific, with frank bleeding seen in a minority of cases, so cases may be mistaken for other, more common diseases or, in the case of Guinea, Lassa fever, which is endemic in the area of the outbreak.[3] Nor are laboratory diagnostics routinely available in West Africa for most viral hemorrhagic fevers.[4] Ebola virus testing of human serum samples collected as far back as 1996 as part of surveillance for Lassa fever in the same region as the current outbreak could help reveal whether humans had exposure to Ebola virus prior to this outbreak.[3] We are presently organizing with collaborators to conduct ELISA antigen testing, PCR, and cell culture for Ebola virus on samples from persons who met the case definition for viral hemorrhagic fever but tested negative for Lassa fever. We will also test all samples for IgG antibody to Ebola virus to explore the prevalence of past exposure.

Could Zaire ebolavirus have been recently introduced into Guinea from Central Africa? Introduction from a human traveler seems unlikely; there is little regular travel or trade between Central Africa and Guinea, and Guéckédou, the remote epicenter and presumed area of first introduction, is far off the beaten path, a minimum 12-hour drive over rough roads from the capitals of Guinea, Liberia, or Sierra Leone (figure 5.1). Furthermore, with the average incubation period as well as time from disease onset until death in fatal cases both a little over a week, a human traveler would have to make the trip from Central Africa to Guéckédou rather rapidly.

If Ebola virus was introduced into Guinea from afar, the more likely traveler was a bat. Although a virus has not yet been isolated, PCR and serologic evidence accumulated over the past decade suggests that fruit bats are the likely reservoir for Ebola virus. The hammer-headed fruit bat (*Hypsignathus monstrosus*), Franquet's epauletted fruit bat (*Epomops franqueti*), and the little collared fruit bat (*Myonycteris torquata*) are among the leading candidates.[5–9] Many of these species are common across sub-Saharan Africa, including in Guinea, and/or may migrate long distances, raising the possibility that one of these wayward flyers may have carried Ebola virus to Guinea.[8] Introduction into humans may have then occurred through exposures related to hunting and consumption of fruit bats, as has been suspected in Ebola virus outbreaks in Gabon.[8] Similar customs have been reported in Guinea, prompting the Guinean government to impose a ban on bat sale and consumption early on in the outbreak.

Field collections and laboratory testing for Ebola viruses of bats collected from the Guinea forest region should shed light on the presence or absence of these various species in the area and possible Ebola virus infection. Indeed, a team of ecologists is already on the ground beginning this work.

But why Guinea and why Guéckédou? Certainly this is not the only place bats migrate. Unfortunately, Ebola virus outbreaks typically constitute yet another health and economic burden to Africa's most disadvantaged populations. Despite the frequently promulgated image of Ebola virus mysteriously and randomly emerging from the forest, the sites of attack are far from random; large hemorrhagic fever virus outbreaks almost invariably occur in areas in which the economy and public health system have been decimated from years of civil conflict or failed development.[10–13] Biological and ecological factors may drive emergence of the virus from the forest, but clearly the sociopolitical landscape dictates where it goes from there—to an isolated case or two or a large and sustained outbreak.

The effect of a stalled economy and government is threefold. First, poverty drives people to expand their range of activities to stay alive, plunging them deeper into the forest to expand the geographic as well as species range of hunted game and to find wood to make charcoal, and deeper into mines to extract minerals, enhancing their risk of exposure to Ebola virus and other zoonotic pathogens in these remote corners. Then, the situation is compounded when the unlucky infected person presents to an impoverished and neglected healthcare facility where a supply of gloves, clean needles, and disinfectants is not a given, leaving patients and healthcare workers alike vulnerable to nosocomial transmission. The cycle is further amplified as persons infected in the hospital return to their homes incubating Ebola virus. This classic pattern was noted in Guinea, where early infection of a healthcare worker in Guéckédou triggered a spread to surrounding prefectures and eventually to the capital, Conakry.[1] Lastly, with an outbreak now coming into full force, inefficient and poorly resourced governments struggle to respond, as we are seeing all too clearly with this outbreak of Ebola virus disease in West Africa, which is now by far the largest on record. The response challenge is compounded in this case by infected persons crossing the highly porous borders of the three implicated countries, requiring intergovernmental coordination, with all the inherent logistical challenges in remote areas with poor infrastructure and communication networks and, in this case, significant language barriers.

Guinea, Liberia, and Sierra Leone, sadly, fit the bill for susceptibility to more severe outbreaks. While the devastating effects of the civil wars in Liberia and Sierra Leone are evident and well documented, readers may be less familiar with the history of Guinea, where decades of inefficient and corrupt government have left the country in a state of stalled or even retrograde development. Guinea is one of the poorest countries in the world, ranking 178 out of 187 countries on the United Nations Development Programme Human Development Index (just behind Liberia [174] and Sierra Leone [177]). More than half of Guineans live below the national poverty line and about 20% live in extreme poverty. The Guinea forest region, traditionally comprised of small and isolated populations of diverse ethnic groups who hold little power and pose little threat to the larger groups closer to the capital, has been habitually neglected, receiving little attention or capital investment. Rather, the region was systematically plundered and the forest decimated by clear-cut logging, leaving the "Guinea forest region" largely deforested (figure 5.3).

The forest region also shares borders with Sierra Leone, Liberia, and Cote d'Ivoire, three countries suffering civil war in recent decades. Consequently, the region has found itself home to tens of thousands of refugees fleeing these conflicts, adding to both the ecologic and economic burden. A United Nations High Commission for Refugees census of camps in the forest region in 2004 registered 59,000 refugees. Although the formal refugee camps have now been dismantled following improved political stability in the surrounding countries, the impact on the region is long-lasting. Having worked in Guinea for a decade (1998–2008) on research projects based very close to the epicenter of the current Ebola virus outbreak, one of the authors (DGB) witnessed this "de-development" first-hand; on every trip back to Guinea, on every long drive from Conakry to the forest region, the infrastructure seemed to be further deteriorated—the once-paved road was worse, the public services less, the prices higher, the forest thinner (figures 5.3 and 5.4).

Guinea fell further into governmental and civil disarray after former president Lansana Conté's death in 2008 left a power vacuum, sparking a series of coup d'états and periods of violence. Although the political situation has now somewhat stabilized, the country struggles to progress;

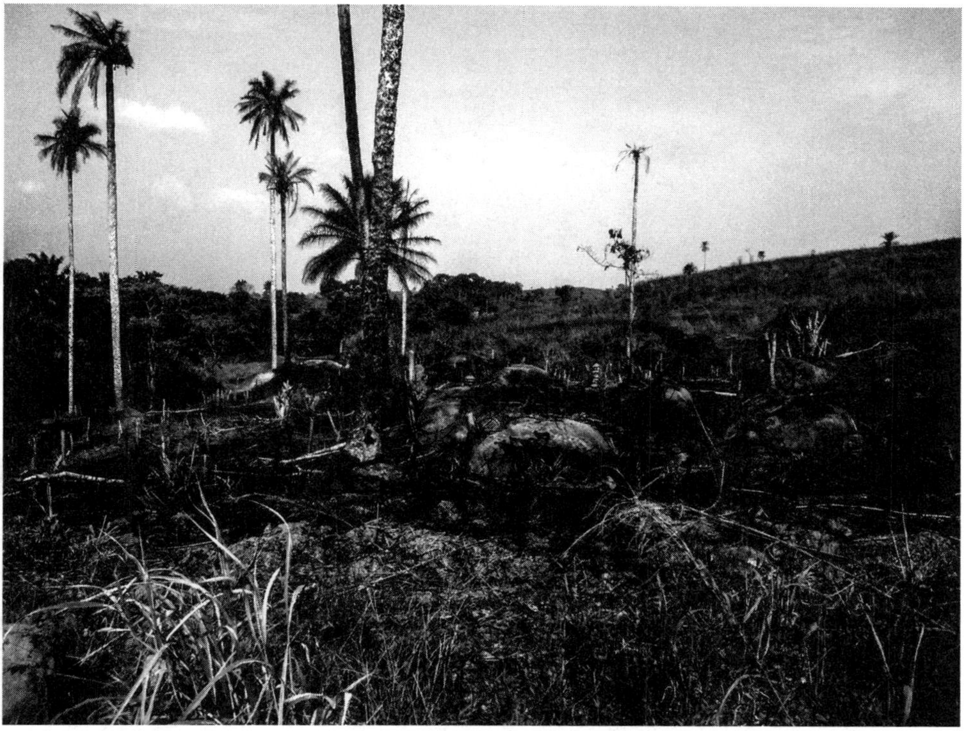

Figure 5.3
The area known as the Guinea forest region, now largely deforested because of logging and clearing and burning of the land for agriculture. Photo credit: Daniel Bausch.

socioeconomic indicators such as life expectancy (56 years) and growth national income (GNI) per capita ($440) have crept up in the past few years, but still remain disparagingly low. Despite a wealth of mineral and other natural resources, Guinea still possesses the eighth lowest GNI per capita in the world, and the incidence of poverty has been steadily increasing since 2003.

Lastly, why is this outbreak of Ebola virus happening now? As best as can be determined, the first case of Ebola virus disease in Guinea occurred in December 2013, at the beginning of the dry season, a finding consistent with observations from other countries that outbreaks often begin during the transition from the rainy to dry seasons.[14–18] Sharply drier conditions at the end of the rainy seasons have been cited as one triggering

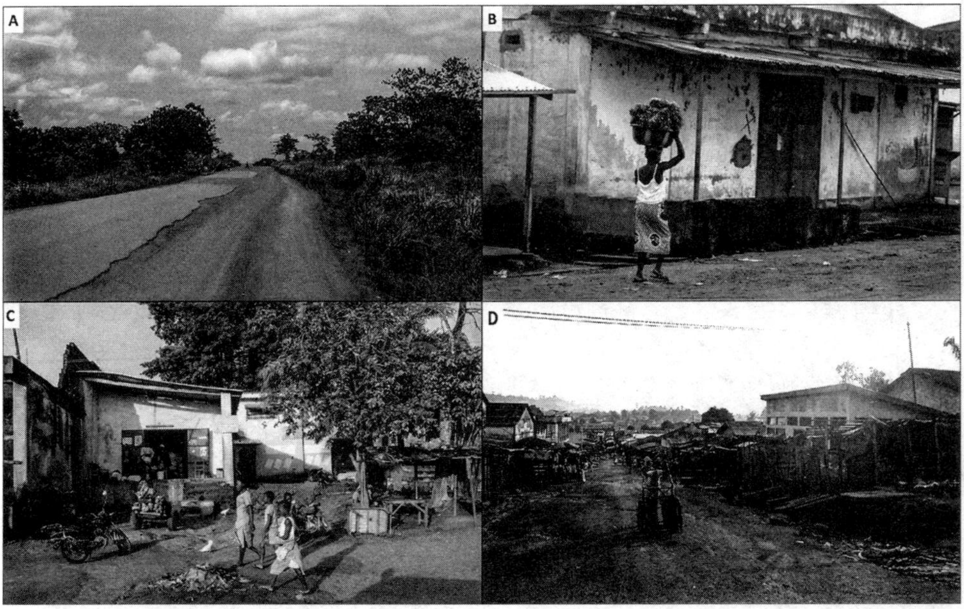

Figure 5.4
Scenes of the degraded infrastructure of the Guinea forest region. (A) Once-paved, but now deteriorated road. (B, C, and D) Street views of the dilapidated town of Guéckédou, the epicenter of the Ebola virus disease outbreak. Photo credit: Frederique Jacquerioz.

event.[17] Although more in-depth analysis of the environmental conditions in Guinea over the period in question remain to be conducted, inhabitants in the region do indeed anecdotally report an exceptionally arid and prolonged dry season, perhaps linked to the extreme deforestation of the area over recent decades. At present, we can only speculate that these drier ecologic conditions somehow influence the number or proportion of Ebola virus–infected bats and/or the frequency of human contact with them.

The precise factors that result in an Ebola virus outbreak remain unknown, but a broad examination of the complex and interwoven ecology and socioeconomics may help us better understand what has already happened and be on the lookout for what might happen next, including determining regions and populations at risk. Although the focus is often on the rapidity and efficacy of the short-term international response, attention to these admittedly challenging underlying factors will be required for long-term prevention and control.

Note

This chapter was originally published in *PLoS Neglected Tropical Diseases* 8, no. 7: e3056, doi: 10.1371/journal.pntd.0003056. Licensed under Creative Commons Attribution (CC BY) license.

Acknowledgments

The authors thank Monica Barrera, Serena Carroll, Barnett Cline, Frederique Jacquerioz, James Mills, Townsend Peterson, Simon Pollett, and Jonathan Towner for creative input and technical support.

Disclaimer

The views expressed in this article are those of the authors and do not necessarily reflect the official policy or position of the World Health Organization, nor the US government.

References

1. Baize, S., D. Pannetier, L. Oestereich, T. Rieger, L. Koivogui, et al. 2014. Emergence of Zaire Ebola Virus Disease in Guinea—Preliminary Report. *New England Journal of Medicine*; E-pub ahead of print. doi:10.1056/NEJMoa1404505.

2. Dudas G, Rambaut A (2104) Phylogenetic Analysis of Guinea 2014 EBOV Ebolavirus Outbreak. PLoS Curr 1: 1–11.

3. Bausch, D. G., A. H. Demby, M. Coulibaly, J. Kanu, A. Goba, et al. 2001. Lassa fever in Guinea: I. Epidemiology of human disease and clinical observations. *Vector Borne and Zoonotic Diseases (Larchmont, N.Y.)* 1:269–281.

4. Khan, S. H., A. Goba, M. Chu, C. Roth, T. Healing, et al. 2008. New opportunities for field research on the pathogenesis and treatment of Lassa fever. *Antiviral Research* 78:103–115.

5. Leroy, E. M., B. Kumulungui, X. Pourrut, P. Rouquet, A. Hassanin, et al. 2005. Fruit bats as reservoirs of Ebola virus. *Nature* 438:575–576.

6. Pourrut, X., A. Delicat, P. E. Rollin, T. G. Ksiazek, J. P. Gonzalez, et al. 2007. Spatial and temporal patterns of Zaire ebolavirus antibody prevalence in the possible reservoir bat species. *Journal of Infectious Diseases* 196 (Suppl 2): S176–S183.

7. Pourrut, X., M. Souris, J. S. Towner, P. E. Rollin, S. T. Nichol, et al. 2009. Large serological survey showing cocirculation of Ebola and Marburg viruses in Gabonese bat populations, and a high seroprevalence of both viruses in Rousettus aegyptiacus. *BMC Infectious Diseases* 9:159.

8. Leroy, E. M., A. Epelboin, V. Mondonge, X. Pourrut, J. P. Gonzalez, et al. 2009. Human Ebola outbreak resulting from direct exposure to fruit bats in Luebo, Democratic Republic of Congo, 2007. *Vector Borne and Zoonotic Diseases (Larchmont, N.Y.)* 9:723–728.

9. Hayman, D. T., P. Emmerich, M. Yu, L. F. Wang, R. Suu-Ire, et al. 2010. Long-term survival of an urban fruit bat seropositive for Ebola and Lagos bat viruses. *PLoS One* 5:e11978.

10. Bausch, D. 2001. Of Sickness Unknown: Death, and Health, in Africa. *United Nations Chronicle* 38:5–13.

11. Bausch, D., and P. Rollin. 2004. Responding to Epidemics of Ebola Hemorrhagic Fever: Progress and Lessons Learned from Recent Outbreaks in Uganda, Gabon, and Congo. *Emerging Infections* 6:35–57.

12. Allan, R. (1998) The progression from endemic to epidemic Lassa fever in war-torn West Africa. In Saluzzo JF, Dodet B, editors. Emergence and Control of Rodent-borne Diseases: Hantaviral and Arenal Diseases. Emerging Diseases 2: 197–205.

13. Bertherat, E., A. Talarmin, and H. Zeller. 1999. Democratic Republic of the Congo: between civil war and the Marburg virus. International Committee of Technical and Scientific Coordination of the Durba Epidemic. *Medecine Tropicale* 59:201–204.

14. Leroy, E. M., P. Rouquet, P. Formenty, S. Souquiere, A. Kilbourne, et al. 2004. Multiple Ebola virus transmission events and rapid decline of central African wildlife. *Science* 303:387–390.

15. Lahm, S. A., M. Kombila, R. Swanepoel, and R. F. Barnes. 2007. Morbidity and mortality of wild animals in relation to outbreaks of Ebola haemorrhagic fever in Gabon, 1994–2003. *Transactions of the Royal Society of Tropical Medicine and Hygiene* 101:64–78.

16. Bermejo, M., J. D. Rodriguez-Teijeiro, G. Illera, A. Barroso, C. Vila, et al. 2006. Ebola outbreak killed 5000 gorillas. *Science* 314:1564.

17. Pinzon, J. E., J. M. Wilson, C. J. Tucker, R. Arthur, P. B. Jahrling, et al. 2004. Trigger events: enviroclimatic coupling of Ebola hemorrhagic fever outbreaks. *American Journal of Tropical Medicine and Hygiene* 71:664–674.

18. Jezek, Z., M. Y. Szczeniowski, J. J. Muyembe-Tamfum, J. B. McCormick, and D. L. Heymann. 1999. Ebola between outbreaks: intensified Ebola hemorrhagic fever surveillance in the Democratic Republic of the Congo, 1981–1985. *Journal of Infectious Diseases* 179 (Suppl 1): S60–S64.

6 Challenges in the Management of the West African Ebola Outbreak

Armand Sprecher

The mention of Ebola prompts thoughts of the archetypal biohazard and difficulty in managing patients with Ebola virus disease (EVD). However, just as difficult to manage are the outbreaks themselves, and this has been true since the discovery of the virus nearly 40 years ago. Past outbreaks have presented a host of difficulties, and many of the challenges of the past were present once more in the recent West African outbreak. However, new problems have arisen that not only present their own challenges, but are synergistic with known past issues. The international public health agencies that have worked in the past to control EVD outbreaks went into this outbreak prepared to deal with the known challenges and work on an outbreak that was of a scale comparable to what has been seen before. The West African outbreak presented challenges we were not prepared for that forced us to scale up, adapt, and respond.

Logistical Challenges in Responding to an Ebola Virus Disease Outbreak

EVD outbreak interventions have always been complex. To respond comprehensively, the international community, in conjunction with local partners, must put into place a wide array of services. To prevent the occurrence of new cases of EVD in areas where confirmed cases have been found, every situation where further transmission might occur needs to be brought under control. To do so, we first need to find people who are infected with Ebola. When these people are alive but sick, we need to transport them safely to a place where they can be cared for safely. When they have already died of the disease, we need to ensure that they are buried safely. When they are infected with the virus but not yet sick, surveillance systems must be put into place to detect these cases as soon as they become ill. Where we have found cases, we need to decontaminate their environment. In communities where Ebola is being transmitted, we engage in health promotion activities to stop behaviors that cause people to become infected. In health care settings, we must reinforce, or sometimes set up where not existent, infection-control procedures to prevent the infection of health care workers or cross-infection of patients who do not yet have EVD. This allows us to safely treat non-Ebola illnesses while remaining vigilant for cases of EVD that might present to these health care settings. While all of this is occurring, epidemiologists are carrying out investigation of the outbreak to determine chains of transmission; anthropologists are studying community beliefs and behaviors that contribute to disease transmission; psychologists are providing mental health support for patients and their families; and special medical services are set up for convalescent EVD patients.

All of these activities are necessary, and if one is absent or underperforming, control of the outbreak suffers. If EVD survivors are not well cared for, new patients will have a disincentive to be identified and brought to the Ebola treatment unit. If the care provided in the treatment units is not humane and of good quality, the word will get out, and patients in the community will have another reason not to be identified. If the anthropologists do not provide insight into local burial traditions and identify areas of compromise so that they may be performed safely while still respecting important rituals, the community will reject the service offered by the burial teams and disease transmission will go on unchecked. Physicians evaluating new arrivals to the Ebola treatment units to determine whether they should be admitted are dependent on the work of the epidemiologists to describe the chains of transmission and risk patterns to make their decision. This interdependency is why a comprehensive set of activities needs to be put into place to control an outbreak.

The Challenge of Geography

Implementing all of the necessary outbreak-control activities in a single location is already manpower-intensive. In each new location where EVD appears, all of the services need to be duplicated if the outbreak is to be controlled. Prior to the West African EVD outbreak, the number of experienced people in the world who could competently launch and supervise these activities was sufficient for one or two instances of a full outbreak-control apparatus. When the outbreak spread from southeastern Guinea to the capital of Conakry, and then to Liberia and Sierra Leone within the first month, four simultaneous outbreak-control operations had to be put into place. In the first month of the outbreak, the available resources were already overstretched.

As each new location drew upon increasingly limited resources, the experienced staff available to respond to the next location rapidly diminished. When the government of Liberia reported cases of Ebola in Monrovia in June of 2014, few experienced people were available to assist the Ministry of Health and Social Welfare when they faced what turned out to be the outbreak's greatest explosion of cases in a single location. The weak support the international community was able to provide to this response may have contributed to the magnitude of the outbreak in Monrovia.

Over the course of the outbreak, dozens of locations across West Africa would require their own outbreak-control activities. The international community responded as quickly as it could, and over the course of the epidemic, thousands of people were trained to carry out various Ebola-control activities. It would be hard to imagine how we might have gone into the West African outbreak with more experienced staff, as EVD was rare and few organizations had interest in maintaining competence to deal with it. However, we might have scaled up sooner, as it was apparent even in that first month that we would be coming up short in the face of what lay ahead. It is not obvious how this might have been done, though. Requests for other organizations to get involved were made repeatedly in the early months of the outbreak,[1,2] but few responded.

A Mobile Population

Scaling up to meet the demands of the unforeseen extension of the outbreak does not address the reason why this was a problem in the first place. Perhaps the most important novelty of the West African Ebola outbreak, and one hallmark which distinguished it from all previous outbreaks, was the mobility of the population.[3] This was the cause of the multiple outbreak metastases that proved to be problematic. Although there had been a small degree of fragmentation of some outbreaks in the past,[4] these had only required control operations to be launched in one or two other locations. Never before had such dispersal of cases occurred. This mobility appears to be the result of the spatial dispersion of friends and family in West Africa, coupled with a transportation infrastructure sufficient to move people about at a cost within the means of much of the population. This made the routine movement of people across several hundreds of kilometers a routine event even before the EVD epidemic. Once people harboring the virus started making similar voyages, cases began to show up in locations well removed from the previously known cases, each requiring yet another set of outbreak-control activities. The resulting strain on resources, most significantly on experienced human resources, was an important factor in allowing the West African outbreak to expand as it did.

Beyond simply taxing resources, the mobile population also posed a challenge for outbreak-control measures as traditionally practiced. When an outbreak is confined to a single region, local teams can keep track of chains of transmission and trace contacts. When cases and contacts move to villages or cities outside the radius of outbreak-control operations, contact is broken. Maintaining surveillance would require knowing the destination of departing cases and contacts and preparing the health authorities there to receive a handoff of responsibility for their follow-up. This was not possible during this outbreak.

A destructive complement to the novel mobility of the affected population was the old problem of our inability to recruit the local population as a partner in outbreak control. We ask people to trust that we have their well-being in mind when we ask the sick to come to the Ebola treatment unit, or when we ask their contacts to allow us to invade their privacy every day for three weeks to see if they become ill or not. If we cannot gain their trust, then our ability to control the outbreak is severely compromised. The fear of Ebola and mistrust of strangers once more in West Africa derailed our attempts to bring the outbreak under control.[5] Patients and their contacts hid, and scared communities let surveillance teams know they were unwelcome. Frightened populations that are also mobile have the option to flee as well, and to go quite some distance when they do.

The naïve response to the problem of a mobile population was to impose restrictions on the movement of people. Several times the governments of West Africa experimented with quarantines, border closures, or "lockdowns." These were of limited effectiveness for several reasons. First, Ebola had usually spread outside of the zones of restriction before the measures were imposed. Second, local communities are often quite adept at circumventing check points and border closures in the parts of the country they inhabit. Finally, oppressive measures are usually counterproductive, as they provide incentive for people to hide from surveillance systems if they think their detection will limit their freedom of movement or that of their family.

In the future, the most effective means of coping with population movement will be to engage individuals' self-interest in remaining close at hand by providing effective medical services. If an effective therapeutic agent becomes licensed for use, its availability in a treatment center will provide a strong reason for a patient or a contact to remain close by. For those cases and contacts that feel the need to move anyway, the availability of a treatment may provide an incentive for them to maintain contact with health authorities. Outbreak-control agencies will still need to develop a means of handover of surveillance for moving cases and contacts.

Risks to Health Care Workers

Despite the difficulties in gaining the trust of the population and carrying out epidemiologic surveillance, patients were nevertheless brought to the treatment units, where another problem awaited: caring for them safely. The iconic image of an EVD outbreak is that of health care workers dressed in their protective gear. The need to protect doctors, nurses, and others working in proximity to Ebola patients has been a feature of outbreak management for decades. It has also been a limitation of their ability to work for just as long. Any material that provides protection from infectious fluids will necessarily reduce evaporative cooling of the body by perspiration. The current configuration of protective clothing can be endured by most people working in the West African environment for about 40 to 60 minutes. Beyond this time limit, the wearer risks heat illness, impaired situational awareness and judgment, and problems with postural stability.[6] At this point, the protective gear becomes a greater liability than it is an asset.

Because of this, a worker no longer represents 8 to 10 man-hours of labor per shift, but rather is limited to 2 to 3 hours of patient contact time. This limitation was more manageable in past outbreaks when the numbers of patients were much lower. The West African outbreak has had more than 50 times the number of cases of the next-largest outbreak on record. More of a problem was the rate at which the number of cases increased, going from less than a hundred new cases per week in July of 2014 to nearly one thousand per week in September of the same year. The demand for care exceeded the ability of the Ebola treatment units to provide it. This disconnect between case incidence and care available led to highly publicized incidents, including the temporary closure to new admissions of the Médecins Sans Frontières facility in Monrovia in September of 2014, and the suspension of intravenous fluid administration until staffing could be suitably expanded.

In the future, if an effective vaccine can provide health care workers with protection, they may be able to wear protective gear that is a good deal more gas-permeable and allows for normal body cooling, and there is reason to believe this is likely.[7] Furthermore, changes that have already been made to the design of Ebola treatment units, such as placement of the entrance to single-patient rooms next to high-risk/low-risk barriers or construction of low-risk corridors with plexiglass walls into larger patient tents, allow limited access to patients from outside of the high-risk zone, so health care workers without protective gear can interact with their patients and carry out some of their patient care tasks unencumbered.

Managerial Limitations

The scale and extension of the outbreak forced into service a great number of people who had no prior experience with Ebola. One of the weaknesses this exposed was the extent to which doctors can be successfully employed as managers. Outbreak-control activities require the coordination and supervision of large numbers of people, many of whom are new to the tasks they are carrying out. An effective manager of Ebola outbreak-control activities needs to determine what is necessary to take care of the current accumulation of tasks as well as the backlog of unaddressed work; to plan a service with sufficient capacity to discharge this work in a timely manner; to request the necessary resources; and to oversee the implementation and running of this service. Medical school does not usually teach these skills. Nevertheless, doctors and epidemiologists are often given responsibility for the management of outbreak-control operations that employ hundreds of people.

For example, contact tracing requires that each person who was in contact with someone ill with Ebola prior to their being taken to the treatment unit be visited each day for twenty-one days from the last contact with the infected individual. A manager of a contact-tracing system needs to be sure that their staff is well trained, has the means to communicate back what they find while they are working, has transportation to allow them to visit each of their contacts, and has sufficient gloves and protection material to safely interact with the contacts they are examining. The manager must be able to review the results of what their teams found each day and be able to motivate them to improve their coverage where gaps are identified. Usually, each case will have 10 to 15 contacts. In a location where one has hundreds of cases, there will be thousands of contacts. Visiting each of these contacts every day requires hundreds of people. Managing contact tracing does not require medical or public health knowledge; it requires excellent organizational and human resource management skills. A doctor may have these by chance. A skilled manager has them by definition. Making managers responsible for the supervision of outbreak-control activities would address the most significant deficiency in this activity.

Contact tracing is but one of the many outbreak-control activities. Each activity needs to be well managed to achieve its objectives. The ensemble of all the interdependent activities is a complex whole which itself needs to be well coordinated. Here again, often at the head of the table at a coordination meeting, we almost always find someone whose professional training has been in medicine and whose experience has not been in coordination of outbreak control, let alone with EVD. Historically, the mandate for outbreak control has been either with persons representing the local ministry of health or with the World Health Organization (WHO). Very rarely in the past have outbreaks been well coordinated by either of these organizations. Past outbreaks have ended despite the coordination of outbreak control rather than because of it. The West African outbreak was no exception.

The managerial shortcomings of the various ministries of health in regard to the coordination of an Ebola response are understandable. They have little experience with EVD, and the West African countries had none. The management skills they need for their usual work can be acquired on the job with ad hoc training where necessary. Management of EVD outbreak-control activities is outside the scope of their normal work. On the other hand, the WHO has been involved in every EVD outbreak since the discovery of the virus, and their mandate is to provide support to the member states in matters such as coordination of outbreak control.

A Failure of International Leadership

Outbreak-control activities are ideally carried out by agencies that are able to do so competently. This does not always occur, but for most outbreak-control activities, experienced external agencies are asked by the local ministry of health to carry out outbreak-control activities because of special skills they possess. Field labs from the Centers for Disease Control and Prevention (CDC) or the Public Health Agency of Canada are given the role of testing blood specimens of suspect patients. Médecins Sans Frontières (MSF) is given responsibility for the care of patients. Epidemiologists from CDC, MSF, WHO, and Epicentre, a satellite agency of MSF dedicated to field epidemiology, carry out outbreak investigation. One would think that an experienced coordinator from WHO would take on the coordination of outbreak control. This, however, almost never happens.

To some extent, this problem stems from the WHO's structure. Article 51 of the WHO's constitution places the authority to respond to the needs of their member states in the hands of the regional offices,[8] which for West Africa is WHO's African Regional Office. However, the part of the WHO that maintains experience with EVD is part of the WHO headquarters in Geneva, Switzerland. Authority and competence are housed in two separate parts of the organization, which have yet to find a way to bridge this divide. The importance of good coordination, and its absence in past outbreaks, has been a well-understood problem for long enough that the failure of the WHO to resolve this issue prior to the West African outbreak makes it one of the more regrettable aspects of this epidemic.[9] Fixing this would take us a long way toward a better response to the next outbreak.

There is some hope that WHO may undertake some of the steps needed to address its problems. An independent expert panel commissioned by WHO to review its response to the EVD outbreak in West Africa noted many of its failings and called for several reforms, including structural ones, noting, "in a Public Health Emergency of International Concern (PHEIC), and possibly in Grade 2 emergencies at the discretion of the Director-General, the reporting lines should switch [away from reporting to the Regional Office]. The regional emergency team and the head of the emergency operation in a country would report directly to the Head of the WHO Centre."[10] It remains to be seen how the WHO will respond.

We went into the West African Ebola outbreak with the same outbreak-control techniques, the same institutions, and, for the most part, with the same people as we went into past outbreaks. In the words of Sean Connery, we brought a knife to a gunfight. As a result, our strengths were out-matched and our weaknesses exposed. The international community scaled up in response. It will be important to go into the next epidemic, not ready to fight the previous war, but instead to apply lessons learned from this outbreak, capitalize on new partnerships, and hold institutions to promises of funding and cooperation.

Notes

1. Médecins Sans Frontières, "Ebola: Massive Deployment Needed to Fight Epidemic in West Africa," press release, June 23, 2014, http://www.doctorswithoutborders.org/news-stories/press-release/ebola-massive-deployment-needed-fight-epidemic-west-africa.

2. James Gallagher, "Ebola Response Lethally Inadequate, Says MSF," BBC News, September 2, 2014, http://www.bbc.com/news/health-29031987.

3. Kathleen A. Alexander, Claire E. Sanderson, Madav Marathe, Bryan L. Lewis, Caitlin M. Rivers, Jeffrey Shaman, et al., "What Factors Might Have Led to the Emergence of Ebola in West Africa?" *PLOS Neglected Tropical Diseases* 9, no. 6 (2015): e0003652, doi: 10.1371/journal.pntd.0003652.

4. Centers for Disease Control and Prevention, "Outbreak of Ebola Hemorrhagic Fever—Uganda, August 2000–January 2001," *Journal of the American Medical Association* 285, no. 8 (2001): 1010–1012, doi: 10.1001/jama.285.8.1010.

5. *The Lancet* editors, "Ebola in West Africa: Gaining Community Trust and Confidence," *The Lancet* 383, no. 9933 (2014): 1946, doi: 10.1016/s0140-6736(14)60938-7.

6. A. G. Sprecher, A. Caluwaerts, M. Draper, H. Feldmann, C. P. Frey, R. H. Funk, et al., "Personal Protective Equipment for Filovirus Epidemics: A Call for Better Evidence," *Journal of Infectious Diseases*, 2015, doi: 10.1093/infdis/jiv153.

7. Ana Maria Henao-Restrepo, Ira M. Longini, Matthias Egger, Natalie E. Dean, W. John Edmunds, Anton Camacho, et al., "Efficacy and Effectiveness of an rVSV-vectored Vaccine Expressing Ebola Surface Glycoprotein: Interim Results from the Guinea Ring Vaccination Cluster-Randomized Trial," *The Lancet* 386, no. 9996 (2015): 857–866, doi: 10.1016/s0140-6736(15)61117-5.

8. World Health Organization, *Constitution of the World Health Organization*, 45th ed., e-book (Geneva: World Health Organization, 2006), http://www.who.int/governance/eb/who_constitution_en.pdf.

9. Kevin Sack, Sheri Fink, Pam Belluck, and Adam Nossiter, "How Ebola Roared Back," *The New York Times*, December 29, 2014, http://www.nytimes.com/2014/12/30/health/how-ebola-roared-back.html.

10. World Health Organization, *Report of the Ebola Interim Assessment Panel*, 1st ed., e-book (Geneva: World Health Organization, 2015), http://who.int/csr/resources/publications/ebola/report-by-panel.pdf.

III The Politics of Ebola

7 What's the Matter Boss, We Sick? A Meditation on Ebola's Origin Stories

Adia Benton

In late October 2014, US President Barack Obama held a press briefing at the White House to describe the US strategy for bringing the 2013–2016 West African Ebola outbreak under control. He said:

> We know that the best way to protect Americans ultimately is going to stop this outbreak at the source. …
>
> And it's critical that we maintain that leadership. The truth is that we're going to have to stay vigilant here at home until we stop the epidemic at its source. …
>
> But what's also critically important is making sure that all the talent, skill, compassion, professionalism, dedication, and experience of our folks here can be deployed to help those countries deal with this outbreak at the source.[1]

Obama's emphasis on "the source" reveals a preoccupation with searching for the origin of the outbreak. Such a search is a deeply human one, in which we "attempt to capture the exact essence of things, their purest possibilities."[2] Anthropologists have written extensively about how people explain misfortune by seeking its source.[3] They go to great lengths to discover the answers to these questions: Who is responsible? Why us? Why now?

Obama, at least officially, located the West African Ebola outbreak's origins in the most affected regions themselves, in order to make a straightforward case for containment "over there" to prevent sickness "over here." This rhetoric operates through a form of projection, where the worst part of ourselves—our most pressing fears—can be displaced and recognized in others. If "health" is perceived to be the normal state of affairs in "the West," then, as anthropologists Jean and John Comaroff have argued, "affliction was taken to be endemic to the life of Africans; it was an unfortunate corollary of their social arrangements, their moral condition, their 'animal ecology.'"[4]

Issues of race cannot be disentangled from projection. Fanon, drawing a connection between projection and anti-blackness, noted that foreignness and evil are attributed to the unknown (black person); when such attributes are identified in oneself, its origins are ascribed to someone else and slated for elimination.[5] Or, to reframe Obama's talking points on Ebola more ominously: It is stopped at its source.

As the outbreak unfolded, origin stories proliferated. Journalists, building on accounts from epidemiologists; residents of Meliandou, Guinea; and survivors, reconstructed a possible scenario of a child playing in a hollowed-out tree where bats lived. From there, they speculated that a single child, the putative "patient zero," became sick. Images of the hollowed-out tree—the alleged "ground zero"—were widely circulated and displayed in popular science press, scientific presentations that I attended, and mainstream media outlets.

Another origin story centered Ebola at the intersections of race, militarization, and the political economy of scientific research. Many West Africans and people of African descent questioned whether the American military–funded laboratory in Kenema, Sierra Leone, and its partners at Tulane University were to blame. They believed scientists working in the lab conducted experiments that put local populations at risk. Like libertarian and right-wing American media sources, they also drew a connection among the region's natural resources, the hemorrhagic viral fever laboratory, and the sketchy presence of the US military's Africa command.[6]

The first lab-confirmed case of Ebola in the United States forced many of us to broaden our vision of what lay at the root of inequitable distribution of quality health care and of Ebola virus disease itself. In early October 2014, while Liberian national Thomas Eric Duncan was being treated for Ebola in a Dallas, Texas, hospital, Liberian president Ellen Johnson Sirleaf apologized to the United States and denigrated Duncan in an interview:

> With the US doing so much to help us fight Ebola ... He's gone there and in a way put some Americans in a state of fear and put them at some risks, so I feel very saddened by that, and very angry with him...
>
> The fact that he knew and he left the country, it's unpardonable, quite frankly. I just hope that nobody else gets infected ... I hope he'll get his treating and then after that they'll send him back and then we'll have to deal with him.

When the reporter asked, "What will you do after he comes home?" Sirleaf laughed and said she would "have to consult with the lawyers."[7]

Sirleaf based her threats on "the fact that he knew," but we can only speculate whether Duncan knew when or where he contracted Ebola. He died on October 8, 2014. We don't know what he knew.

A week after Duncan's death, Sierra Leone hosted the United States Agency for International Development chief administrator, Rajiv Shah, to discuss the Ebola response. The communications unit for Sierra Leone's president, Ernest Bai Koroma, issued a press release entitled: "'We Will Not Export Ebola' President Koroma Assures." The message was clear: Koroma, like Sirleaf, was also deeply concerned with ensuring that citizens from his country did not spread Ebola to Americans.[8]

The two leaders' statements were upsetting. Why had they felt the need to assert their concern for Americans' health? Why did they identify so strongly with the Americans? Why did they couch their concern for these distant others within the context of aid? Their remarks, which registered as unreciprocated identification with Americans' "plight," resonated with Malcolm X's ideas about a psychological disposition borne of chattel slavery. Speaking on the difference between the "house negro" and the "field negro," Malcolm X said:

> When the master would be sick, the house Negro identified himself so much with his master he'd say, "What's the matter boss, we sick?" His master's pain was his pain. And it hurt him more for his master to be sick than for him to be sick himself.[9]

Here, Malcolm X outlines how identification with the master class is intimately linked to a division of labor and relationships of exploitation ordered along spatial and racial lines. Feelings of allegiance and identification with elites among a managerial class, Malcolm X suggests, are forged under conditions of violence that uphold terms of their servitude, their presumed inferiority, their eagerness to accept what they are given, in exchange for meager personal gain. As a kind of managerial class, the "house negro" builds an uneasy intimacy with elites and, for his survival, depends on the remains of his master's spoils. He eats the scraps from his master's table, lives in his master's attic, and wears his master's old clothes. The managerial class strongly identifies with the master class, yet recognize they will never be fully incorporated into it. The burdens of this relationship are deeply felt by the masses; they both witness and experience the structural, symbolic, and psychological violence this relationship engenders.

In short, we sick.

The presidential statements about their concern for Americans take for granted a political and economic relationship that is pathological, even pathogenic. This relationship has long devalued and destabilized the infrastructure necessary—systems, staff, and stuff[10]—to prevent and contain a disease like Ebola. The three countries hardest hit by the outbreak are largely dependent on foreign assistance to finance their health systems. Some money for "public" health care never becomes part of government health budgets and is instead funneled through international NGOs who are, in turn, financed by development agencies mostly in the West.

It is easy to blame civil war for the crumbling health systems in Liberia and Sierra Leone. Indeed, many doctors, nurses, and technicians left Liberia and Sierra Leone during the war. Health facilities fell into disrepair or were destroyed, along with the infrastructure for monitoring and training clinicians and public health specialists.[11] Yet structural adjustment programs of the 1980s had already had a significant impact on the health systems in these countries, well before there was a civil war.[12] As in many poor countries around the world, the terms of World Bank and International Monetary Fund loans that accompanied structural adjustment reforms required countries like Liberia and Sierra Leone to roll back social services, devalue their currencies, and increase exports of cash crops with low tariffs.[13] The end of African socialism in Guinea in 1984 also marked a sharp decline in the national health system, with only short-lived improvements in health indicators after the institution of the cost-recovery primary health care scheme (also known as the Bamako Initiative) in 1988.[14]

As Sierra Leonean political scientist Fodei Batty reminds us, the Ebola virus has followed the path of the civil war.[15] The region where the war began has also been the site of an ongoing, century-long land grab. In Liberia, Firestone ushered in a new way of doing business in the 1920s;[16] a pattern of exploitation persisted through the war in the 1990s, with the company turning away its Liberian employees to be slaughtered by the rebels and paying "protection" money to Charles Taylor to ensure smooth operations.[17] Although it built an Ebola ward in April 2014 to respond to a single case on the plantation, Firestone refused nonemployees treatment until early August—even as government and NGO-sponsored treatment units filled to capacity outside the plantation's borders.[18] But we can push the clock back even farther: Predatory practices of commodity extraction have economically devastated the region since the trans-Atlantic slave trade.[19]

Today, African presidents like Koroma and Sirleaf manage the extraction and export of natural resources and distribute the revenues these exports generate. In an attempt to attract foreign investors, Sierra Leone provides tax breaks to international mining and agribusiness companies that have diminished the resources required to administer public services like health care and education.[20]

Ebola disrupted this system and substituted it with its own viral economy. In July and August 2014, mining and agribusiness companies and international NGOs, which offer services usually provided by the public sector, evacuated their staff. An expanded emergency aid industrial complex built up around the Ebola response filled the economic gap left by suspended bauxite, diamonds, and rutile extraction operations and long-term development initiatives. The Ebola aid coming into the three countries was under intense scrutiny, as international and local media outlets, accountability watchdog agencies, and citizens demanded more precise accounting. Some saw a persistent lack of accountability as contributing to failures to contain the epidemic, with some going as far to suggest that better accountability measures for Ebola constituted a cure.[21] But as Marilyn Strathern has argued, accountancy and accountability are not the same—nor does the former remediate an enduring legacy of extraction, dependency, and exploitation.[22] A true "reckoning" of Ebola response—a different origin story—must also account for failures to implement robust public health systems in light of extensive and significant health-sector expenditure by foreign donors in the aftermath of the civil conflicts in these countries.

As Sirleaf and Koroma intimated during their apologies and assurances to Americans, the disruption of extraction, cultivation, and export of commodities gave rise to fears that Ebola would become a primary export to the West. The local elites were no longer comfortable in their position of managing resource extraction and allocation; of distributing aid flows to other elites; and of allowing international NGOs to conduct the parallel business of making live and letting die. In the wake of Ebola, leaders of these three countries were under pressure to prove their capacity to manage the virus and control its movements.

It is bitterly ironic, then, that Koroma and Sirleaf felt the need to publicly express their concern for the health and welfare of Americans, a group that, at the time and to this day, has not experienced an Ebola epidemic. They have demonstrated, however, the lengths they are willing to go, the extent to which they will try to exercise sovereign power over the living, by establishing *cordons sanitaires* around entire regions and communities, instituting national lockdowns, and supporting village-based quarantines.[23] None of these are innately bad interventions. But these leaders' inability to manage the Ebola crisis at home threatened their political legitimacy on many fronts.[24] They risked losing whatever credibility they had with their trading partners. Their failure to care for the multitudes of sick people threatened their political power at home.[25]

We sick.

By the time Duncan succumbed to his illness, Sirleaf's popularity had declined.[26] She was unpopular in Monrovia before the outbreak, but a confrontation between residents of West Point, an informal settlement in Monrovia, and national security forces signaled a turning point. This community has a history of civil conflict, dispossession and marginalization, and unsubstantiated rumors had circulated about the government wanting to clear slum housing for urban development.[27] When area residents opposed the establishment of an isolation unit for outsiders in their community, the military quarantined West Point. Already tense relations between the government and area residents were stretched to the breaking point. During the quarantine, troops fired shots into crowds of protestors, killing a 15-year-old boy and injuring others.

In some ways, Koroma has been more successful than Sirleaf in asserting his authority, but he has also been criticized for those to whom he has entrusted leadership positions. In 2012, he appointed Miatta Kargbo, a pharmaceutical representative, to the post of minister of health and sanitation. Allegedly the relative of a close friend, she became the object of scorn during this outbreak when she appeared before Sierra Leone's Parliament and mocked two health care workers who succumbed to Ebola.[28] A video in which she accused the health care workers of adultery circulated as evidence of her incompetence and lack of integrity. That it took so long to replace her with someone more experienced did not help Koroma's cause.[29]

When Martin Salia, a Sierra Leonean surgeon with permanent resident status in the United States, succumbed to Ebola in Nebraska, many asked: Why are Africans the only people to have died from Ebola in the United States? What was the message to be communicated to the rest of the world by these deaths? For them, a global hierarchy of value had been erected along fault lines of class, race, nationality, and region. The technologies of surveillance, monitoring, and exclusion began not at airports in New York, Newark, Atlanta, Chicago, and Washington, DC. Rather, the barriers to passage to the United States are erected at the ports of Conakry, Monrovia, and Freetown. The barriers to quality health care in the United States were racialized and located in "the clinic" itself. The problem of infection is reified and policed by West African leaders themselves, who have expressed an internalized disregard for their own afflicted as they also extended unreciprocated sympathy for the "pre-afflicted" in the United States.

We sick.

Origin stories have profound consequences for how people explain, interpret, and respond to an emergent Ebola crisis. They also impact how we begin to plan for "the next one," an important concern as the West African epidemic dies down. Experts have rekindled security paradigms of public health, which are premised on thinking not only of diseases as global threats that transgress national borders, but of certain places (and their residents) as posing inherent danger to others.[30] The accounts presented in this chapter suggest the need for multiple origin stories attentive to political economy and its intersections with race, class, and scientific knowledge production. We must *imagine* new origin stories. If imagination signals a present future, then memory serves, as Barbara Adam has noted,[31] as a kind of "past future," in which origin stories about the current epidemic—and efforts to end it—must also be understood within the context of enduring histories of exploitation, deception, dependency, and re/source extraction.

Acknowledgments

For their editorial assistance with earlier versions of this essay, I would like to thank Aaron Bady at The New Inquiry, where a different version was originally published, and Siddhartha Mitter.

Notes

1. Remarks by President Obama on Ebola, October 28, 2014, https://www.whitehouse.gov/the-press-office/2014/10/28/remarks-president-ebola.

2. Michel Foucault, *The Foucault Reader* (New York, Pantheon, 1984), 78.

3. For the most canonical example for the discipline of anthropology, see E. E. Evans-Pritchard, *Witchcraft, Oracles and Magic Among the Azande* (Oxford: Oxford University Press, 1937).

4. Jean Comaroff and John L. Comaroff, *Of Revelation and Revolution, Vol. 2: The Dialectics of Modernity on a South African Frontier* (Chicago: University of Chicago Press, 1991), 336. This is relevant for interpreting visual imagery used in news reporting about the Ebola outbreak that drew on old racial tropes, like those described by Dionne and Seay in this volume.

5. Frantz Fanon, *Black Skin, White Masks* (New York: Grove Press, 1967), 190.

6. Aaron Klein, "Military's Ebola Mission: Edge Out China in Africa?" *World News Daily*, October 12, 2014, http://www.wnd.com/2014/10/militarys-ebola-mission-to-edge-out-china-in-africa/.

7. Adrienne Arsenault, "Liberia's Ellen Johnson Sirleaf Says Ebola Was like 'Unknown Enemy,'" *CBC News*, October 2, 2014, http://www.cbc.ca/news/world/liberia-s-ellen-johnson-sirleaf-says-ebola-was-like-unknown-enemy-1.2785503.

8. "We Will Not Export Ebola—President Koroma Assures," press release issued by the Sierra Leone presidential communications office, October 16, 2014.

9. Malcolm X, "Malcolm Describes the Difference between the 'House Negro' and the 'Field Negro'" (lecture, Michigan State University, East Lansing, MI, January 23, 1963), http://ccnmtl.columbia.edu/projects/mmt/mxp/speeches/mxt17.html.

10. Paul Farmer, "Diary: Ebola," *London Review of Books,* October 23, 2014, 36: 38–39, http://www.lrb.co.uk/v36/n20/paul-farmer/diary.

11. Angel Desai and Muctarr Jalloh, "Sierra Leone's Long Recovery from the Scars of War," *Bulletin of the World Health Organization,* no. 88 (2010): 725–6, http://www.who.int/bulletin/volumes/88/10/10-031010/en/.

12. Carol P. MacCormack, "Primary health care in Sierra Leone," *Social Science & Medicine* 19, no. 3 (1984): 199–208.

13. Alexander Kentikelenis, Lawrence King, Martin McKee, and David Stuckler, "The International Monetary Fund and the Ebola Outbreak," *The Lancet Global Health* 3, no. 2 (2014): e69–70, http://www.thelancet.com/article/S2214109X14703778/fulltext.

14. Daniel Levy-Bruhl, Agnes Soucat, Raimi Osseni, Jean-Michel Ndiaye, Boubacar Dieng, Xavier de Bethune, et al., "The Bamako Initiative in Benin and Guinea: Improving the Effectiveness of Primary Health Care," *The International Journal of Health Planning and Management* 12, no. S1 (1997): S49–S79.

15. Fodei Batty, "Reinventing 'Others' in a Time of Ebola," Hot Spots: Cultural Anthropology Online, October 7, 2014, http://www.culanth.org/fieldsights/589-reinventing-others-in-a-time-of-ebola.

16. W. E. B. Du Bois, "Liberia, the League and the United States," Foreign Affairs 11 (1933): 682–95, https://www.foreignaffairs.com/articles/liberia/1933-07-01/liberia-league-and-united-states.

17. Christian T. Miller and Jonathan Jones, *Firestone and the Warlord: The Untold Story of Firestone, Charles Taylor and the Tragedy of Liberia* (New York: ProPublica, 2014).

18. Claire Zillman, "In Africa, Foreign Corporations Protect Their Own from Ebola," *Fortune,* August 8, 2014, http://fortune.com/2014/08/08/africa-ebola-corporations. Curiously, stories about Firestone's competency and generosity as a company proliferated in mainstream media—US National Public Radio, *Forbes* and other news outlets in early October 2014—effectively erasing any doubts raised in early August about their role in combating the epidemic.

19. Joseph E. Inokori and Stanley L. Engerman, eds., *The Atlantic Slave Trade: Effects on Economies, Societies and Peoples in Africa, the Americas, and Europe* (Durham, NC: Duke University Press, 1992).

20. Provost, Claire, "Sierra Leone Tax Breaks Put Foreign Investment Ahead of Poor, Say NGOs," *The Guardian,* April 15, 2014, http://www.theguardian.com/global-development/2014/apr/15/sierra-leone-tax-incentives-foreign-investment-before-poor-ngos. The article refers to a consulting report by Mark Curtis, "Losing out: Sierra Leone's Massive Revenue Losses from Tax Incentives," Christian Aid UK, 2014, http://www.christianaid.org.uk/images/Sierra-Leone-Report-tax-incentives-080414.pdf.

21. "UK MPs Urge Strict Accountability for Ebola Funds," *Ghana Web Health News,* October 8, 2014, http://www.ghanaweb.com/GhanaHomePage/health/artikel.php?ID=329352.

22. Marilyn Strathern, "'Improving Ratings': Audit in the British University System," *European Review (1997)* 5, no 3 (1997): 305–21, http://journals.cambridge.org/abstract_S1062798700002660.

23. Adam Nossiter, "Lockdown Begins in Sierra Leone to Battle Ebola," *New York Times,* September 19, 2014, http://www.nytimes.com/2014/09/20/world/africa/ebola-outbreak.html. Compare with a later account by Umaru Fofana, "Ebola

Outbreak: Sierra Leone in Lockdown," *BBC News*, March 27, 2015, http://www.bbc.com/news/world-africa-32083363.

24. Theresa Ammann, "Ebola in Liberia: A Threat to Human Security and Peace," Hot Spots: Cultural Anthropology Online, October 7, 2014, http://www.culanth.org/fieldsights/597-ebola-in-liberia-a-threat-to-human-security-and-peace.

25. Patricia Jabbeh Wesley, "Liberia's Ebola Epidemic: Did the Government Fall Asleep at the Wheel?," Hot Spots: Cultural Anthropology Online, October 7, 2014, http://www.culanth.org/fieldsights/602-liberia-s-ebola-epidemic-did-the-government-fall-asleep-at-the-wheel.

26. Ibid.

27. Marcus S. Zoleh, "No Plan to Demolish West Point, Says Commissioner Flowers," *The Informer* (Monrovia), February 6, 2013, http://accessliberia.com/no-plan-to-demolish-west-point-says-commissioner-flowers/.

28. "Health Minister Miatta Kargbo Mocks Nurse Who Died of Ebola," *Awareness Times* (Freetown), June 18, 2014, http://news.sl/drwebsite/publish/article_200525604.shtml.

29. "Health Minister Miatta Kargbo Sacked," *The Sierra Leone Telegraph* (Freetown), August 29, 2014, http://www.thesierraleonetelegraph.com/?p=7208.

30. David L. Heymann, Lincoln Chen, Keizo Takemi, David P. Fidler, Jordan W. Tappero, Mathew J. Thomas, et al. "Global Health Security: The Wider Lessons from the West African Ebola Virus Disease Epidemic," *The Lancet* 385 (2015): 1884–1901, http://www.thelancet.com/article/S0140673615608583/fulltext. See also Ilona Kickbusch, James Orbinski, Theodor Winkler, and Albrecht Schnabel, "We Need a Sustainable Development Goal 18 on Global Health Security," *The Lancet* 385 (2015): 1069, http://www.ncbi.nlm.nih.gov/pubmed/25797551.

31. Barbara Adam, "Of Timescapes, Futurescapes and Timeprints," lecture, Luneburg University, Luneburg, Germany, June 17, 2008.

8 American Perceptions of Africa during an Ebola Outbreak

Kim Yi Dionne and Laura Seay

The cover of an August 2014 issue of *Newsweek* featured an image of a chimpanzee behind the words, "A Back Door for Ebola: Smuggled Bushmeat Could Spark a U.S. Epidemic." There was virtually no chance that "smuggled bushmeat" would bring Ebola virus disease (EVD) to America. Far from presenting a legitimate public health concern, the authors of the story and the editorial decision to use chimpanzee imagery on the cover placed *Newsweek* squarely in the center of a long and ugly tradition of treating Africans as savage animals and the African continent as a dirty, diseased place to be feared. Reactions to the recent EVD outbreak in the United States highlight longstanding ethnocentric and xenophobic popular understandings of Africa.

The 2013–2016 EVD outbreak in West Africa was unique in many respects. It was by far the largest recorded outbreak of the disease, infecting at least 28,000 individuals and killing over 11,000.[1] It was also the first time that EVD spread beyond the African continent, with a traveler, Thomas Eric Duncan, bringing the virus to the United States, where two of the hospital staff who cared for him—nurses Nina Pham and Amber Vinson—were infected. Likewise, during this epidemic, various health care professionals were treated for the virus in Europe and the United States. In the United States, hysteria characterized much of the public reaction to EVD's spread across the Atlantic. Although EVD was never a threat to the general public, sales of hand sanitizer and cleaning products spiked,[2] children relocating from nonaffected African countries were kept out of school,[3] and politicians responded to public fears with threats of quarantining all health workers returning from the infection zone, regardless of their actual exposure to Ebola virus.[4]

In this chapter, we seek to explain the hysterical, irrational public response to EVD in the West, primarily in America. In chapters 2 and 6 of this volume, respectively, Patricia Henwood and Armand Sprecher examined the international response in terms of supporting interventions against EVD in West Africa. In chapter 3, Michael Connor Jr. described the EVD cases treated in the West, while Marjorie Kruvand discusses the activities of hospitals dealing with the diagnosis of EVD inside the United States in chapter 11. Our chapter puts the *Newsweek* cover story and similar episodes during the 2013–2016 outbreak in a broader context of how Africa is viewed in the West and how these perceptions can shape response to a public health epidemic. We use a "College 101" approach to chronicle the domestic American response to the 2013–2016 EVD outbreak, covering some of the basics: history, geography, psychology, and our own discipline, political science. We conclude with a discussion of the implications of xenophobic responses in the West to public health epidemics in Africa.

History: A Long Tradition of Categorizing Africans and Immigrants as Inferior and Diseased

The Europeans who colonized Africa in the late nineteenth century were members of a culture obsessed with classifying and categorizing the natural world. This quest built much of modern biology, but also led to unscientific justifications for the colonial project. One idea developed by Frederick Coombs expounded the then-popular theory of phrenology: that the size, shape, and other physical characteristics of a person's skull determine one's intelligence (among other traits).[5] The notion that physical characteristics of the skull determined intelligence, capability, and skill was patently false, but Europeans like Coombs worked hard to find evidence for their claims, starting with the assumption that they—white, northern and Western Europeans—were the smartest and therefore the characteristics of their own skulls were evidence of superior traits.

It followed from this assumption that southern Europeans (who were not considered to be racially "white" at the time) and people of color were inherently less intelligent than northern and western Europeans with light-colored skin.[6] Victorian phrenologists developed elaborate typologies supposedly showing that Africans had the most apelike—and therefore most "savage"—skull types. The Victorians thus concluded Africans were less intelligent than northern Europeans and in need of the "civilizing mission" that colonization was supposed to bring, thus justifying African subjugation under colonial rule.[7]

While Coombs's book may be the best known of the works of Victorian phrenology, the racism that his conjectures embodied was deeply embedded in the culture of colonizing states. Most Westerners of the time believed that people of color were "savages," desperately in need of the benefits of modernity, Christianity, and intelligence that the colonists believed they were well suited to bring to Africa.[8]

As societal norms tend to do, the racism embodied in the notion that African people's skulls are more similar to those of other primates than those of *Homo sapiens* skulls made its way into popular culture. And it did so in a particularly insidious way: by portraying Africans as apelike savages. Images showing Africans as apelike were commonplace. In popular culture, people of African origin were portrayed in postcards, film, and literature as "savages" who were not as "civilized" as their colonizers.[9] These stereotypes even extended to children's books. A Belgian cartoon book, *Tintin au Congo,* is perhaps the most famous of these representations; there, the Congolese people whom the boy adventurer Tintin encounters are at times almost indistinguishable from the great apes of central Africa. Similarly, Africans with exaggerated lips and other features who maintain extended-limb, apelike postures are portrayed throughout the original texts of the Babar series.[10]

As historian Sarah Steinbock-Pratt notes, imagery of Africans as hypersexualized savages—cannibals, even—persisted in cinematic representations of Africa throughout the twentieth century.[11] For example, early volumes of *Tarzan of the Apes*, a wildly popular book series, stereotyped Africans as cannibalistic threats to "civilized" society.[12] This long history of white people associating Africans with primates—both savage, running wild in the jungle (never mind that most Africans live nowhere near a jungle or any of the great apes), and threatening any white people who approach—has not evolved much in the last century.

In American society, there has been a persistent association of immigrants and disease.[13] The Immigration Act of 1891 explicitly excluded from entry to the United States all "persons suffering from a loathsome or dangerous contagious disease."[14] Even before the Immigration Act of 1891 passed, immigrants were often scapegoats for infectious disease. For example, in the 1870s, San Francisco's Chinatown was considered a "laboratory of infection," and whenever a major epidemic threatened the city, "health officials descended upon Chinatown with a vengeance."[15]

Associating immigrants with disease has continued in the century since the US Immigration Act of 1891. In 1991 Haitian refugees who tested positive for HIV were "confined like prisoners" at the naval base at Guantanamo Bay—despite knowledge at least five years earlier that HIV was not transmitted via casual contact.[16] Early narratives about AIDS in the United States often invoked Haitians as a major "at-risk" population and the pathway through which HIV made its way from Africa to North America; these beliefs stemmed from underlying racist, ethnocentric attitudes.[17] Likewise, in the 2003 SARS epidemic, New York City's Chinatown was identified as a site of contagion and risk despite never having a single case of SARS.[18]

International migration has historically been associated with transporting disease, and metaphors of plague and infection have been used to marginalize and exclude diaspora communities.[19] The aforementioned American episodes of overreaction to public health threats linked in the public imagination to immigrants—particularly nonwhite immigrants—have their equivalents in Canada,[20] Australia,[21] and elsewhere in the Western world.[22]

Geography: Africa as Monolithic

Despite the vastness of the African continent, historical mapping norms, particularly the Mercator projection, make Africa appear to be about the same size as Greenland, which is actually about one-fourteenth the size of the African continent. Misunderstandings about the continent have been perpetrated by old maps alongside cultural and media norms that often refer to Africa as one entity rather than an 11.7 million-square-mile land mass comprised of 54 countries and more than 1.1 billion people who speak over 2,000 different languages. The combined landmasses of the United States (including Alaska), Europe, and China are all smaller than the African continent.[23] The United States would fit into Africa three times.

When a dangerous disease like EVD breaks out, Americans who are used to referring to "Africa" as one entity will mistake just how big of a threat

EVD actually is, who might have been exposed to it, and the likelihood of infection. One example of a failure to appreciate the size of Africa and the distance between different African countries was the response to a woman vomiting on a flight from New York to Los Angeles in October 2014. Tens of firefighters and paramedics, along with airport police, county health officials, and FBI agents were on the scene at LAX to greet the plane and vomiting passenger.[24] Why the huge response? She had been to Africa. It turns out she had not been to one of the most affected countries in West Africa but had been to South Africa—and she had airsickness, not a viral hemorrhagic fever. The distance between Liberia, the westernmost point of the main outbreak zone, and South Africa is over 3,000 miles. Yet the knowledge that the woman had simply been on the African continent was enough to terrify the flight crew and first responders into the unreasonable and unwarranted assumption that she might actually have been infected with EVD.

Of 54 African countries, only three countries had widespread and intense transmission of EVD. The three countries most heavily affected in the 2013–2016 Ebola outbreak were Guinea, Liberia, and Sierra Leone; more than 99 percent of recorded cases were in these three countries.[25] Although there were also cases in Senegal, Nigeria, and Mali, these outbreaks were classified as having "localized transmission," and EVD was contained relatively quickly in these countries.[26] Considering the case of the sick air passenger traveling from South Africa, as we see in the map in figure 8.1, South Africa is almost as far from the outbreak zone as you can get while still being in Africa.

The American traveling from South Africa was only one example of overreaction in the United States. A Brooklyn teenager who had traveled from Sudan was ill with flu-like symptoms when New York health authorities thought he might have been exposed to Ebola virus.[27] The map shows how incredibly far away Sudan is from the outbreak zone—more than 2,500 miles. Moreover, air travel from one African country to another—especially outside of each region—is difficult, and most commercial airlines had canceled flights into and out of airports in the outbreak zone. Someone needing to travel from Liberia to Sudan would have to transit via another country—probably in Europe or the Middle East—to get there, and the expense and difficulty of such travel, coupled with enhanced screening procedures for passengers originating from the outbreak zone, made it

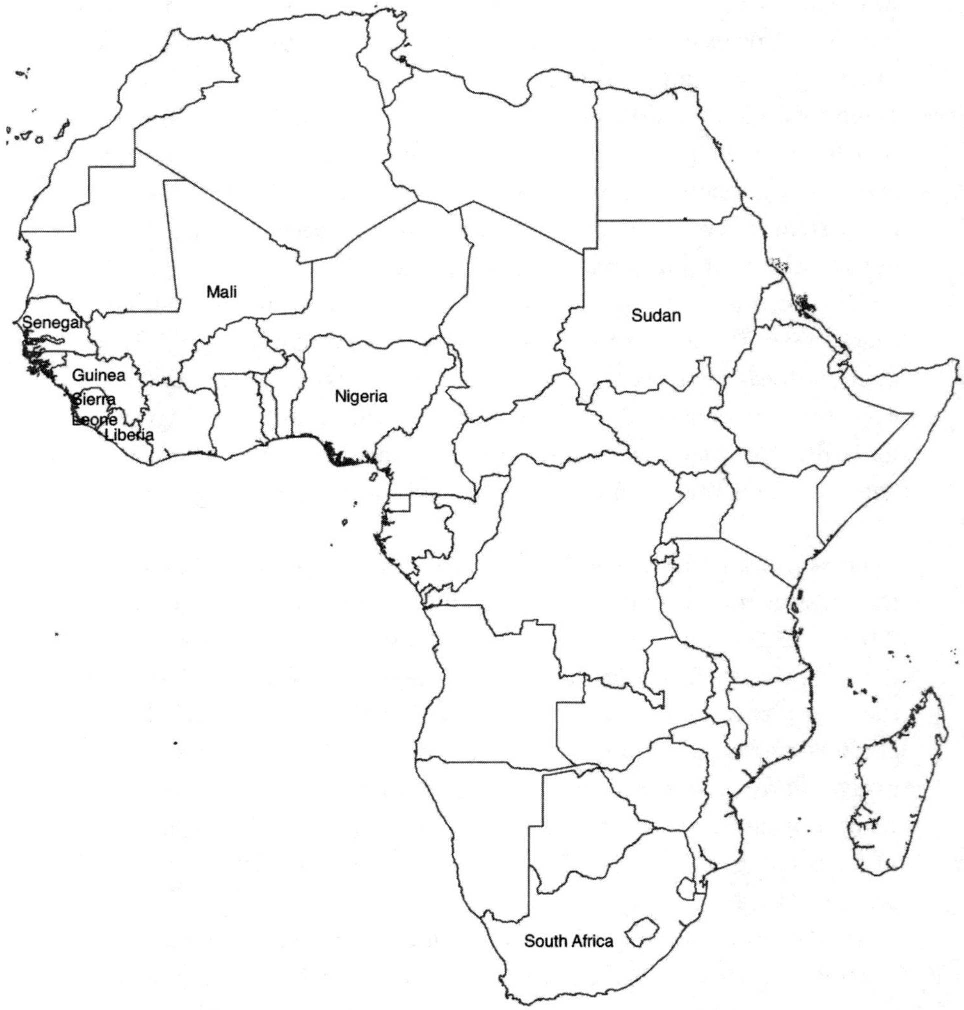

Figure 8.1
West African countries with Ebola cases in the 2013–2016 outbreak are identified, as are South Africa and Sudan, to show the great distance between these two countries and the center of the epidemic.

extremely improbable that someone would be infected with EVD in a place like Sudan.

As if the loss of life weren't enough, the negative effects of the lack of geographic knowledge about Africa in this crisis had and continue to have real and negative economic impacts for Africans whose countries and lives are untouched by EVD. Estimates of the economic damage caused by EVD in this outbreak are as high as $32.6 billion.[28] But the outbreak wrought havoc on African economies beyond the three most heavily affected by EVD, and that damage was completely avoidable. For example, bookings for safaris in East and Southern Africa—including for the famed Great Migration in Kenya and Tanzania—plummeted due to the EVD outbreak. In a survey of 500 safari tour operators, a majority of respondents had a decrease in bookings and an increase in cancellations in the wake of the West African Ebola outbreak.[29]

Psychology: How We Think about a Place or a People Shapes How We Respond

Fearmongering narratives about EVD circulating in the popular media have had a serious effect on how people think about the disease. Although the risk of contracting EVD was near zero in the United States, there was great public concern about a potential EVD outbreak on American soil. Nationally representative public opinion polls found 39–52 percent of Americans—depending on the date of the poll—thought there would be a large EVD outbreak in the United States, and more than a quarter of Americans were concerned that they or someone in their immediate family would get sick with EVD in the year following their survey interview.[30] These surveys, and others taken during the height of hysteria in the United States, show that Americans grossly overestimated their risk of infection.[31]

Beyond overestimation of risk, the *Newsweek* story and similar media reports suggested increased vulnerability to EVD in the United States. The potential for an American outbreak raised emotions like anxiety, fear, and disgust, and these emotions sometimes influence policy preferences and prejudice.[32] Under increased anxiety, Americans usually increase their support for policies that fight contagion, often at the risk of curbing civil liberties.[33] Additionally, contexts of increased vulnerability will likely amplify negative reactions to people heuristically associated with disease.[34] In the case of the *Newsweek* story, the many African migrants living in the Bronx (and potentially elsewhere in the United States) accused of liking bushmeat are further marginalized. The negative reactions to increased vulnerability include having more xenophobic attitudes. A study conducted in the wake of an outbreak of avian influenza showed that germ aversion was associated with support of exclusionary immigration attitudes and that perceived threat of the avian flu outbreak was associated with support for health-based immigration criteria.[35]

The *Newsweek* story likely generated additional prejudice against African migrants, a population that already suffers from greater prejudice than other immigrant groups. In a study predating the Ebola outbreak, researchers found that simply manipulating the geographical origin of a hypothetical immigrant group—from Eastern Africa to Eastern Asia to Eastern Europe—yielded significant differences in attitudes in a study population toward the immigrant group.[36] Relatedly, a recent review of public attitudes toward immigration points out how prejudice and ethnocentrism can engender support for more restrictive immigration attitudes.[37]

Political Science: Politicking during an Epidemic

The peak of Ebola panic occurred during the thick of a US political campaign period. In addition to lower-profile state and local races, midterm Congressional elections took place in November 2014, as did elections for the governorship of 36 states. Faced with a relatively uninformed and inexperienced public when it came to Ebola, the outbreak was ripe for political exploitation. One prominent example was retired physician and then-US representative from the state of Georgia Phil Gingrey, who wrote a letter to the Centers for Disease Control and Prevention director regarding his concerns that migrant children crossing into the United States from Mexico were likely carrying EVD—as well as other "deadly diseases" that are "not indigenous to this country."[38]

Numerous American politicians took full advantage of the Ebola panic to fearmonger in hopes of boosting their and their parties' electoral success. Roughly 20 percent of over 1,600 e-newsletter communications from members of Congress in the period before the elections called attention to Ebola, which was twice as much as was communicated about other popular issues like Obamacare and immigration; 82 percent of e-newsletter communications mentioning Ebola were from Republicans.[39] Excluding references made in the media to President Barack Obama, Republicans also produced twice as much media coverage as Democrats in US news articles about EVD.[40] Analysts saw politicizing the outbreak as part of the Republicans' midterm elections strategy.[41] Once the midterm elections were over, media coverage of EVD dropped dramatically.[42]

Public opinion polls conducted during the outbreak reflected these partisan patterns. Survey respondents in a nationally representative poll taken in September—before Thomas Eric Duncan was diagnosed with EVD—showed strong partisan differences in how the United States should respond to the outbreak in West Africa. Only 37 percent of Republicans thought the United States should send financial aid, compared to 49 percent of Democrats.[43] There was a similar gap between Republicans and Democrats for sending medical supplies (78 percent vs. 91 percent), sending medical personnel to train and assist doctors (58 percent vs. 68 percent), sending troops to assist with enforcing quarantines (9 percent vs. 21 percent), and in investing more money in Ebola research (60 percent vs. 68 percent).[44] After Thomas Eric Duncan's diagnosis and the infections of nurses Nina Pham and Amber Vinson, the gap between partisan Americans' opinions about the Ebola outbreak widened. In a mid-October 2014 poll, 72 percent of Republicans thought the United States wasn't doing enough to contain the EVD outbreak, compared to only 48 percent of Democrats who felt the same way.[45] The partisan divide was also sharp in attitudes about potential policy responses; for instance, more Republicans (74 percent) than Democrats (46 percent) felt the US government should ban all direct flights from Africa.[46]

Even when public opinion is a partisan mirror of political elites' behavior and opinions, it is challenging to substantiate that politicians making public statements about Ebola influenced citizens' opinions about Ebola, because it could be that politicians are simply advocating on behalf of the opinions of their constituents. However, there is some evidence that politicization of the EVD outbreak increased negative attitudes toward immigrants. In survey experiments conducted among Americans in November and December 2014, the politicization of EVD by political elites negatively affected public opinion on immigration. More specifically, a single statement criticizing the Obama administration's response to Ebola increased anti-immigrant attitudes by six percentage points.[47]

Conclusion

Coombs, the Victorians, and the people who created appalling twentieth century popular culture relating to Africa were engaging in a practice called "othering."[48] Othering happens when an in-group (in this case, white northern Europeans) treats other groups of people (the out-group—here, Africans and other people of color) as though there is something wrong with them by identifying perceived "flaws" in the out-group's appearance, practice, or norms. The "unhealthy" are often othered and stigmatized.[49] Research conducted both under laboratory settings[50] and during actual disease outbreaks[51] shows an association between disease salience and negativity toward foreigners. Although individual characteristics such as perceived vulnerability to disease and ideological beliefs about group hierarchies facilitate perceptions of disease threat as located among out-groups, othering is also dependent on media context and pre-existing representations of out-groups.[52] Thus, portrayals of Africa and Africans in the media—whether during an outbreak or beforehand—are critically important in shaping whether Africans will be othered during disease outbreaks.

Othering has real consequences. Othering is particularly harmful in the context of a health epidemic because it "hampers the containment of contagion during an infectious epidemic by compelling people to reject public health instructions."[53] Scholars have reported on the racist and ethnocentric othering of Africans in the time of AIDS.[54] But othering during a public health scare is not directed only at Africans, as the SARS epidemic clearly illustrated.[55] Likewise, international media othering of African events or issues is not limited to infectious disease outbreaks, but also occurs in reporting on conflict. Othering of Somalia in the early 1990s led to the misidentification and oversimplification of the conflict's dynamics by global policy actors, which led to two decades of misguided and ineffective policy responses to the Somalia crisis.[56] *Newsweek*'s use of a chimpanzee to represent a scientifically invalid story about an African disease is a classic case of othering. It suggests that African immigrants are to be feared, and that apes—and African immigrants who might eat them—could bring a deadly disease to the pristine shores of the United States of America.

The long history of associating immigrants and disease in America and the problematic impact that association has on attitudes toward immigrants should make us sensitive to the impact of the "othering" of African immigrants to the United States during the 2013–2016 EVD outbreak in West Africa. Fearmongering about infinitesimally small risks in a given context serves no purpose to the greater good of trying to curb disease transmission and relieve people's suffering in another context.

Acknowledgments

Portions of this chapter were previously published as posts on The Monkey Cage, a blog about political science and politics at *The Washington Post* and as a brief commentary in a special symposium on Ebola published by *PS: Political Science and Politics*. We are grateful to Adia Benton, Ruxandra Paul, Ken Sherrill, two anonymous reviewers, and the editors of this volume for their comments.

Notes

1. Data current as of March 24, 2016. See Centers for Disease Control and Prevention, "2014 Ebola Outbreak in West Africa—Case Counts," Centers for Disease Control and Prevention, accessed March 27, 2016, http://www.cdc.gov/vhf/ebola/outbreaks/2014-west-africa/case-counts.html.

2. Rheana Murray, "The Ebola Effect: Schools Shut Down, Sanitizer Sales Spike," ABC News, last modified October 16, 2014, http://abcnews.go.com/Business/ebola-effect-schools-shut-sanitizer-sales-spike/story?id=26247311.

3. Alex Napoliello, "Ebola anxiety keeps African students from attending N.J. school," NJ.com, October 20, 2014, http://www.nj.com/burlington/index.ssf/2014/10/amid_ebola_fears_students_from_africa_kept_home_in_south_jersey.html.

4. Brady Dennis, Lena H. Sun, and Mark Berman, "N.Y., N.J., Illinois to Impose New Ebola Quarantine Rules," *Washington Post*, October 25, 2014, http://www.washingtonpost.com/national/health-science/ny-nj-governors-impose-new-ebola-quarantine-rules/2014/10/24/8096e43e-5bac-11e4-8264-deed989ae9a2_story.html; Kaci Hickox, "Caught Between Civil Liberties and Public Safety Fears: Personal Reflections from a Healthcare Provider Treating Ebola," *Journal of Health & Biomedical Law* 11 (2015): 9–23.

5. Frederick Coombs, *Coombs' Popular Phrenology: Exhibiting the Exact Phrenological Admeasurements of Above Fifty Distinguished and Extraordinary Personages, of Both Sexes with Skulls of the Various Nations of the World* (Boston: Coombs, 1841).

6. Patrick Brantlinger, "Victorians and Africans: The Genealogy of the Myth of the Dark Continent," *Critical Inquiry* 12, no. 1 (1985): 166–203.

7. Ibid.

8. Ibid.; Padre Antonio Vieira, 'Children of God's Fire': A Seventeenth-Century Jesuit Finds Benefits in Slavery but Chastises Masters for their Brutality in a Sermon to the Black Brotherhood of Our Lady of the Rosary," ed. Robert Conrad, *Children of God's Fire: A Documentary History of Black Slavery in Brazil* (University Park, PA: Pennsylvania State University Press, 1994), 163–73; Mort Rosenblum, *Mission to Civilize: The French Way* (New York: Harcourt, 1986).

9. Joseph Conrad, *Heart of Darkness* (1899/1902); Wayne Martin Mellinger, "Postcards from the Edge of the Color Line: Images of African Americans in Popular Culture, 1893–1917," *Symbolic Interaction* 15, no. 4 (1992): 413–33; Sarah Steinbock-Pratt, "The Lions in the Jungle: Representations of Africa and Africans in American Cinema," in *Africans and the Politics of Popular Culture*, eds. Toyin Falola and Augustine Agwuele (Rochester, NY: University of Rochester Press, 2009), 214–36.

10. Stephen O'Harrow, "Babar and the Mission Civilisatrice: Colonialism and the Biography of a Mythical Elephant," *Biography* 22, no. 1 (1999): 86–103; blot, "'Tintin au Congo' ou la mission civilisatrice de la colonization," Samarra, UN Blog Mondomix, November 28, 2009, http://blogs.mondomix.com/samarra.php/2009/11/28/tintin-au-congo-ou-la-mission-civilisatr.

11. Steinbock-Pratt, "The Lions in the Jungle."

12. Jeff Burgland, "Write, Right, White, Rite: Literacy, Imperialism, Race, and Cannibalism in Edgar Rice Burroughs' *Tarzan of the Apes*," *Studies in American Fiction* 27, no. 1 (1999): 53–76.

13. Howard Markel and Alexandra Minna Stern, "The Foreignness of Germs: The Persistent Association of Immigrants and Disease in American Society," *The Milbank Quarterly* 80, no. 4 (2002): 757–88.

14. Immigration Act of 1891, 51st Congress, 2nd session, *Congressional Record* 551 (March 3, 1891): 1084–86.

15. Joan Trauner, "The Chinese as Medical Scapegoats in San Francisco, 1870-1905," *California History* 57, no. 1 (1978): 70–87.

16. George Annas, "Detention of HIV-Positive Haitians at Guantánamo," *The New England Journal of Medicine* 329, no. 8 (1993): 589–92.

17. Paul Farmer, *AIDS and Accusation: Haiti and the Geography of Blame* (Berkeley, CA: University of California Press, 1992).

18. Laura Eichelberger, "SARS and New York's Chinatown: The Politics of Risk and Blame during an Epidemic of Fear," *Social Science & Medicine* 65, no. 6 (2007): 1284–95.

19. Ian Harper and Parvathi Raman, "Less Than Human? Diaspora, Disease and the Question of Citizenship," *International Migration* 46, no. 5 (2008): 3–26.

20. Svetlana Reitmanova, "'Disease-Breeders' among Us: Deconstructing Race and Ethnicity as Risk Factors of Immigrant Ill Health," *Journal of Medical Humanities* 30, no. 3 (2009): 183–90.

21. Alison Bashford, "At the Border: Contagion, Immigration, Nation," *Australian Historical Studies* 33, no. 120 (2002): 344–58.

22. John Welshman and Alison Bashford, "Tuberculosis, Migration, and Medical Examination," *Journal of Epidemiology and Community Health* 60, no. 4 (2006): 282–84.

23. Deborah Smith Johnston and Barbara Brown, "Curriculum Guide: How Big is Africa?" *African Studies Center, Boston University*, 1998, http://www.bu.edu/africa/outreach/resources/curriculum/curriculum-guide/.

24. Willian Avila and Kate Larsen, "Sick Passenger Causes Ebola Scare at LAX," *NBC Southern California,* October 12, 2014, http://www.nbclosangeles.com/news/local/Possible-Ebola-Case-Reported-at-LAX-Sunday-278955751.html.

25. World Health Organization, "Ebola Situation Report," World Health Organization, May 20, 2015, http://apps.who.int/ebola/en/current-situation/ebola-situation-report-20-may-2015.

26. A few cases were also reported beyond the African continent—one each in Italy, Spain, and the United Kingdom and four in the United States. World Health Organization, "Ebola Situation Report," May 20, 2015.

27. CBS New York, "Another Possible Ebola Scare In NYC As New Screenings Start At JFK," October 11, 2014, http://newyork.cbslocal.com/2014/10/11/another-possible-ebola-scare-in-nyc-as-new-screenings-start-at-jfk/.

28. Mark Roland Thomas, Gregory Smith, Francisco H. G. Ferreira, David Evans, Maryla Maliszewska, Marcio Cruz, et al., "The Economic Impact of Ebola on Sub-Saharan Africa: Updated Estimates for 2015," World Bank, January 20, 2015, http://www-wds.worldbank.org/external/default/WDSContentServer/WDSP/IB/2015/01/19/000112742_20150119170232/Rendered/PDF/937210REVISED000Jan02002015000FINAL.pdf.

29. Jeroen Beekwilder, "The Unfortunate Impact of the Ebola Outbreak on the Safari Industry," *SafariBookings.com,* September 24, 2014, https://www.safaribookings.com/blog/180.

30. Harvard School of Public Health, "Ebola Poll Topline," August 20, 2014, http://cdn1.sph.harvard.edu/wp-content/uploads/sites/21/2014/08/ebola_Topline_final_08-20-14.pdf; Harvard School of Public Health, "Ebola Poll II Topline,"

October 15, 2014, https://cdn1.sph.harvard.edu/wp-content/uploads/sites/21/2014/10/Ebola-II_Topline_15-October-2014_final.pdf.

31. See also YouGov, "*The Economist*/YouGov Poll," October 11–13, 2014, https://d25d2506sfb94s.cloudfront.net/cumulus_uploads/document/09julkfx4i/econTabReport.pdf.

32. Logan Casey, "Emotions and the Politics of Ebola," *PS: Political Science and Politics* 48, no. 1 (2015): 7–8.

33. Bethany Albertson and Shana Gadarian, " Ebola, Anxiety, and Public Support for Protective Policies," *PS: Political Science and Politics* 48, no. 1 (2015): 8–9.

34. Jason Faulkner, Mark Schaller, Justin H. Park, and Lesley A. Duncan, "Evolved Disease-Avoidance Mechanisms and Contemporary Xenophobic Attitudes," *Group Processes & Intergroup Relations* 7, no. 4 (2004): 333–53.

35. Eva G.T. Green, Franciska Krings, Christian Staerklé, Adrian Bangerter, Alain Clémence, Pascal Wagner-Egger, et al., "Keeping the Vermin Out: Perceived Disease Threat and Ideological Orientations as Predictors of Exclusionary Immigration Attitudes," *Journal of Community and Applied Social Psychology*, 20 (2010): 299–316.

36. Faulkner et al., "Evolved Disease-Avoidance," 333–53.

37. Jens Hainmueller and Daniel J. Hopkins, "Public Attitudes toward Immigration," *Annual Review of Political Science* 17 (2014): 225–49.

38. Phil Gingrey, "Letter to Thomas R. Frieden, Director of Centers for Disease Control and Prevention," July 7, 2014, https://docs.google.com/file/d/0B_KEK8-LWmzhLXI2OU0yTFFyRTg/edit.

39. Lindsey Cormack, "The Ebola outbreak generated greater response from Republican lawmakers," The Monkey Cage blog, *Washington Post,* November 14, 2014, http://www.washingtonpost.com/blogs/monkey-cage/wp/2014/11/14/the-ebola-outbreak-generated-greater-response-from-republican-lawmakers/.

40. Mark Daku and Kim Yi Dionne, "'The ISIS of Biological Agents': Media Coverage of Ebola in the United States." Paper presented at the International Conference on Public Policy, Milan, Italy, July 2, 2015.

41. Jeremy W. Peters, "Cry of G.O.P. in Campaign: All Is Dismal," *New York Times,* October 9, 2014, http://www.nytimes.com/2014/10/10/us/politics/republican-strategy-midterm-elections.html; Matt Gertz and Rob Savillo, "Report: Ebola Coverage on TV News Plummeted after Midterms," *Media Matters for America,* November 19. 2014, http://mediamatters.org/research/2014/11/19/report-ebola-coverage-on-tv-news-plummeted-afte/201619.

42. Gertz and Savillo, "Report: Ebola Coverage."

43. The question asked, "Do you think the United States should or should not take each of the following actions to combat the Ebola outbreak in West Africa? Send financial aid." YouGov, September 13–15, 2014. "*The Economist*/YouGov Poll."

44. YouGov, September 13–15, 2014. "*The Economist*/YouGov Poll."

45. The question asked, "Do you think the United States is doing enough, too much, or not enough to contain the Ebola outbreak?" YouGov, October 18–20, 2014. "*The Economist*/YouGov Poll."

46. The question asked, "Do you think the US government should/should not ban all direct flights from Africa?" *The Economist*/YouGov Poll, October 18–20, 2014.

47. Claire Adida, Kim Yi Dionne, and Melina Platas Izama, "Ebola, Elections, and Immigration: Experimental Evidence of Disease Threat Shaping Attitudes toward Immigrants," unpublished working paper, University of California-San Diego, Smith College, and Stanford University, 2015.

48. Lois Weis, "Identity Formation and the Processes of 'Othering': Unraveling Sexual Threads," *Educational Foundations* 9, no. 1 (1995): 17–33.

49. Robert Crawford, "The Boundaries of the Self and the Unhealthy Other: Reflections on Health, Culture and AIDS," *Social Science & Medicine* 38, no. 10 (1994): 1347–65.

50. Faulkner et al., "Evolved Disease-Avoidance," 333–53.

51. Franciska Krings, Eva G. T. Green, Adrian Bangerter, Christian Staerklé, Alain Clemence, Pascal Wagner-Egger, et al., "Preventing Contagion with Avian Influenza: Disease Salience, Attitudes toward Foreigners, and Avoidance Beliefs," *Journal of Applied Social Psychology* 42, no. 6 (2012): 1451–66.

52. Ingrid Gilles, Adrian Bangerter, Alain Clémence, Eva G.T. Green, Franciska Krings, Audrey Mouton, et al., "Collective Symbolic Coping with Disease Threat and Othering: A Case Study of Avian Influenza," *British Journal of Social Psychology* 52, no. 1 (2013): 83–102.

53. Eichelberger, "SARS."

54. Sydney Bryn Austin, "AIDS and Africa: United States Media and Racist Fantasy," *Cultural Critique* no. 14 (1989): 129–52.

55. Eichelberger, "SARS"; Peter Washer, "Representations of SARS in the British Newspapers," *Social Science & Medicine* 59, no. 12 (2004): 2651–71.

56. Catherine Besteman, "Representing Violence and 'Othering' Somalia," *Cultural Anthropology* 11, no. 1 (1996): 120–33.

9 The Ebola Sentinel: A Legal Analysis of US Pandemic Preparedness

Alexandra L. Phelan

It was not until August 8, 2014—four months after identification of the first probable cross-border spread from Guinea to Liberia—that the World Health Organization (WHO) director-general, Margaret Chan, convened an emergency committee and declared the outbreak of Ebola virus disease (EVD) in West Africa a public health emergency of international concern (PHEIC). The declaration of a PHEIC has particular status under international law. Firstly, it indicates that an epidemic constitutes a sufficient public health risk to other countries through the international spread of the disease, ideally driving WHO member states to provide technical and financial assistance to control and prevent the spread of the outbreak. Secondly, a PHEIC enables the director-general to issue nonbinding temporary recommendations advising countries of the health measures they should—or should not—take in responding to the infectious disease outbreak.

Accompanying the declaration of the PHEIC were temporary recommendations advising non-West African countries against implementing international travel or trade restrictions. In particular, Director-General Chan advised against visa bans and increased screenings at airports for people traveling from West Africa, except for actual EVD cases and their contacts. In addition, she reiterated the importance of respecting civil liberties in implementing any health measures.

The WHO director-general's powers to respond to a potential PHEIC are contained within the International Health Regulations (2005) (IHR). Revised after the 2002–2003 SARS outbreak, the IHR aim to prevent, detect, and control the international spread of infectious disease while ensuring that countries do not take measures that unnecessarily interfere with international travel and trade. Unlike other international laws that require countries to sign and ratify a treaty for it to be legally binding, the IHR are automatically binding upon WHO member states—including the United States.[1]

While the WHO's delay in declaring a PHEIC has been widely criticized, it parallels the limited attention the outbreak was receiving in developed countries, including the United States. While only on the other side of the Atlantic Ocean, the political and media coverage in the United States of the Ebola outbreak in West Africa was limited until July 2014, when two American health care workers were infected and repatriated to the United States for medical treatment.

The US response to the 2013–2016 EVD outbreak provides salient lessons on the state of pandemic preparedness of US political and legal systems. Only four cases were diagnosed within the United States,[2] yet EVD is the sentinel that has demonstrated that US pandemic preparedness is not necessarily a question of whether the law is adequate, but rather how incorrectly used legal powers and conflicts between federal and state priorities can hamper the legal frameworks that aim to protect the public's health.

This chapter examines three instances that exemplify the Ebola sentinel in US public health legal preparedness: 1) border closures; 2) border screenings; and 3) quarantine and isolation measures. The chapter then briefly considers possible solutions to the gaps in the US pandemic preparedness legal response.

Foundations of United States Public Health Law

The US Constitution is the supreme law of the United States of America. The scope of the public health powers at all levels of US government—federal, state, and local—are limited by protections of fundamental civil liberties under the Constitution. Under the Fourth and Fourteenth Amendments, neither the federal nor state governments may deprive a person of their life, liberty, or property without the due process of the law—meaning access to a fair, orderly, and just judicial procedure. The Constitution grants express powers to the federal government, concurrent powers held by both the federal and state governments, and powers reserved solely for the states. This division forms the primary basis for the complexities of the US public health legal regime.

The primary source of the federal government's public health power is derived from its exclusive powers to regulate commerce between states and with foreign nations under the Commerce Clause.[3] This gives the federal government the power to make laws with respect to preventing and controlling the spread of infectious diseases between states or from foreign countries into the United States.[4] In contrast, states derive their law-making powers for public health from their inherent "police powers" and reserved under the Tenth Amendment to the Constitution. States' police powers enable them to regulate behavior and enforce order within their territory for the protection and maintenance of the health, safety, or welfare of their citizens. This broad power forms the legal legitimacy for states to take measures for public health or to delegate aspects of their public health police powers to local governments, as well as to request assistance from federal authorities.

A Legal Analysis of US Responses to Ebola

International borders are the traditional legal boundaries of a nation's sovereignty and were therefore the logical focus of many public health measures and laws aimed at preventing the spread of Ebola into and within the United States.

Border Closures

Despite the WHO director-general's temporary recommendations to the contrary, a number of countries unaffected by Ebola implemented border closure measures.[5] On October 8, 2014, 27 Members of Congress—including three Democrats—wrote to President Obama requesting that the State Department impose a travel ban on citizens of Liberia, Sierra Leone, and Guinea until the end of the outbreak.[6] The requested travel ban included suspension of visas already issued and denying entry to the United States. The authors of the letter called on President Obama not to "pass the buck" to the WHO, "an organization of unelected bureaucrats and political appointees of foreign countries" with "no duty to protect the lives and well-being of Americans."[7] In response, President Obama released a video message to the nation, urging Americans not to "give into hysteria or fear," noting that "trying to seal off an entire region of the world—were that even possible—could actually make the situation worse."[8]

Border closures are protectionist measures from long-gone, pre-globalization eras with limited effectiveness that have the potential to impede the supply of medical necessities and trained health care workers to most-affected regions.[9] In addition, visa bans may result in potentially infected individuals changing their travel strategies in an attempt to evade border controls, undermining public health measures.[10] In a globalized world, such actions risk increasing the likelihood of the international spread of infectious disease. While the epicenter of the 2013–2016 EVD outbreak remained in the West African region, it was pivotal to ensure that vital food and medical supplies as well as trained health care workers were able to travel to affected areas. Travel bans resulted in commercial airlines reducing or ceasing flights, hampering the flow of aid and health care workers to the region, raising concerns that health care workers would not volunteer to assist given fears that they would not be able to return to the United States after working with patients with EVD.[11] The call for President Obama to close US borders in response to the outbreak demonstrates how domestic legal power and authority may conflict with international regimes. While the president had the domestic legal power to enact such bans (through the State Department and Department of Homeland Security), such measures would likely breach the United States's legal obligations under the IHR.[12] This was indeed the case for both Australia and Canada, which breached their obligations under the IHR when they imposed visa bans for nations with widespread and persistent Ebola transmission, namely Liberia, Guinea, and Sierra Leone.[13] Despite these breaches, there is currently no enforcement regime—such as legal sanctions—beyond international political pressure to hold countries accountable for breaches of IHR obligations.[14]

Border Screenings

Following the identification of the first imported Ebola case into the United States in October 2014 (Mr. Thomas Duncan), the Centers for Disease Control and Prevention (CDC) and the United States Department of Homeland Security's Customs and Border Protection (CBP) commenced enhanced entry screening at five major US airports: New York's JFK and Newark International Airports, Dulles International Airport in Washington, DC, Hartsfield-Jackson Atlanta International Airport, and Chicago O'Hare International Airport.[15] These five airports were estimated to handle 94 percent of all travelers to the United States who had recently been in Guinea, Liberia, or Sierra Leone.[16] Upon arrival from these countries, CBP officers screened travelers with questions about symptoms and any potential exposure to Ebola, as well as checked their temperature using noncontact thermometers and conducted visual observations of other Ebola symptoms. If an individual self-reported or measured a fever or other symptoms, or if they had been in a situation where exposure may have occurred, CPD referred the person to CDC public health officers at the airport for further assessment (discussed below). These noninvasive screening methods are permissible health measures at points of entry under the IHR and legitimate public health measures under domestic law.[17]

Despite this, the effectiveness of border screening in identifying possible EVD cases was limited, as it relied on infected individuals either exhibiting symptoms or self-declaring possible exposures to EVD. For example, even if border screening had been in place, it is possible that they would not have detected Mr. Duncan's illness, as he was not exhibiting symptoms and may have been unaware of or chosen not to self-declare potential exposures.[18] The most valuable opportunity border screening provided was the provision of education and establishing active monitoring for cases that subsequently developed in the United States, such as New York doctor Craig Spencer.[19] It is important to note, however, that as a medical doctor who had worked with EVD patients in Guinea, it is likely that border screening was not necessary for effective monitoring and follow-up for Dr. Spencer.[20] Despite the immense cost, border screening may be used as a political tool to reassure the public that the government is in control of the disease. However, the limited effectiveness of border screening in detecting EVD cases ultimately undermined any reassurance such measures gave to the public.[21] For future infectious disease outbreaks, the use of border screening measures—while legally available and perhaps politically preferable—must be carefully tailored, with the realistic limits of the process communicated to the public so as to not undermine broader public health efforts.

Quarantine and Isolation

While often used interchangeably—including in public health legislation—quarantine and isolation technically reference separate health strategies.[22] Quarantine involves restricting the movement of individuals who have been exposed, or potentially exposed, to infectious disease during its period of communicability during the incubation period.[23] Isolation, however, is the separation of individuals known to be infected—determined through testing and physical examination—for the period of communicability.[24] A range of legal powers exists for quarantine and isolation in the United States, from local governments—acting with delegated state power—to the federal jurisdiction. While the constitutionality of these powers have been affirmed over the course of more than a century, the 2013–2016 EVD epidemic demonstrated the ease by which such powers can become politicized, revealing possible future weaknesses in the use of quarantine and isolation powers during an infectious disease outbreak (see chapter 16 for a detailed analysis).

Unlike other federations,[25] the United States federal government does not have an express constitutional power to make laws with respect to quarantine and isolation. Rather, the Constitution's Commerce Clause empowers the US Secretary of Health and Human Services, under the Public Health Services Act, to take measures to prevent the entry and spread of communicable diseases between states and from foreign nations into the United States.[26] The day-to-day operation of this power is delegated to the CDC, which can authorize quarantine and isolation measures to prevent the introduction, transmission, and spread of certain communicable diseases into the United States from foreign countries[27]—or to prevent the spread of certain communicable diseases from one state into another, including where the CDC believes that measures taken by a state are insufficient.[28] These measures apply only to certain communicable diseases as determined by an executive order of the president, including Ebola.[29] The CDC does not typically use its federal authority for quarantine, however, historically leaving decisions on individual quarantines to states.[30]

Within their respective territories, states have the general authority under their police powers to enact public health measures, including quarantines.[31] The exact content of quarantine powers is determined by state legislation. As a result, there is significant variance between states in the scope and procedures for imposing quarantine, including in some instances delegation of quarantine powers to local public health authorities.

Despite this authority, states are bound by the Fourteenth Amendment to the US Constitution to ensure the individuals subjected to the exercise of quarantine powers are provided with due process—both procedurally and substantively—and ensure equal protection through their nondiscriminatory application. As a result, given the significant limitations on an individual's liberty, the proper execution of quarantine powers must satisfy substantive due process tests,[32] including the requirement that quarantine be "reasonable."[33] However, more than a century of public health law and federal CDC guidelines that may help define "reasonableness" risk being ignored by the executive or legislative branches of government when politics, misinformation, and infectious disease mix.

During the 2013–2016 EVD outbreak, the CDC issued detailed guidelines on public health measures states and local authorities should take in identifying and monitoring possible EVD cases, which—even in high risk cases—did not recommend the use of traditional quarantines. Table 9.1 sets out key aspects of the CDC's recommended health measures, implemented with the assistance of the CBP, for asymptomatic individuals.[34]

Despite the detail of these guidelines, a number of states ignored the CDC and Department of Homeland Security guidelines and procedures and used their legal powers to impose their own quarantine procedures.[35] Over the course of October and November, state government officials in California,[36] Connecticut,[37] Florida,[38] Georgia,[39] Illinois,[40] Maine,[41] Maryland,[42] New Jersey,[43] and New York[44] announced policies of varying degrees, but all exceeded the federal CDC guidelines. In New York and New Jersey, mandatory 21-day quarantines were imposed for health care workers returning from countries with intense EVD transmission, who would typically fall under the CDC's "some risk" category.[45]

On October 24, 2014, nurse Kaci Hickox returned to the United States after working for Médecins Sans Frontières in Sierra Leone. According to court documents,[46] upon her arrival at Newark Airport, New Jersey, Ms. Hickox was detained, and despite an initial temperature check showing no elevated temperature and clearance from the CDC, the New Jersey Department of Public Health (DPH) placed Ms. Hickox under mandatory, involuntary quarantine through the use of an Administrative Public Health Order, issued at the discretion of the New Jersey state's DPH. As an asymptomatic health care worker with only some risk of exposure, these measures appear to exceed the CDC's guidelines and may have amounted to an unreasonable exercise of the state's legal powers. Three days later, Ms. Hickox was released and allowed to travel to her home state of Maine. Unlike in New Jersey, under Maine state law quarantine orders must be issued by a court.[47] The commissioner of the Maine DPH applied for a court order to impose a

Table 9.1

CDC Recommended health measures for asymptomatic individuals during the 2013–2016 EVD outbreak

Exposure category	Included individuals	Public health measures required
High risk	• direct exposure to blood or bodily fluids of a symptomatic Ebola patient without appropriate PPE (such as through needle stick injury, splashes to eyes, nose, or mouth, or bodily fluids directly on skin. • direct contact with a dead body without appropriate PPE in an intense transmission country (Liberia, Guinea, Sierra Leone). • lived in the same household and provided direct care to a symptomatic patient deemed to be at high risk of infection	• direct active monitoring (daily fever and symptom monitoring through direct observation). • no travel on public or long-distance transport. • self-exclusion from public gatherings and the workplace. • quarantine not required: non-congregate activities permitted provided a 3-foot distance from other people kept (e.g., jogging in a park).
Some risk	• direct contact with a symptomatic patient in an intense transmission country while wearing PPE (e.g. as health care workers)	• direct active monitoring • any restrictions on movement to be assessed, on a case-by-case basis while still allowing non-congregate public activities with a 3-foot distance.
Low (but not zero) risk	• brief direct contact, without appropriate PPE, with person with EVD in the early stages of the disease. • brief proximity to person with EVD without appropriate PPE	• travelers: active monitoring (daily fever and symptom monitoring without direct observation) • health care workers: direct active monitoring • No further restrictions.
No identifiable risk	• contact with asymptomatic Ebola patient or their contacts • potential exposure to EVD more than 21 days previously • travelers in countries without widespread EVD transmission	No restrictions

mandatory quarantine order on Ms. Hickox. The Maine District Court rejected the application for a mandatory quarantine on the grounds that the state had not met its burden of proof that such a measure was necessary, but upheld the requirement for direct active monitoring (consistent with the CDC's guidelines).[48] As the differences in these two states demonstrate, the legal authority to order a quarantine can have a significant impact, with the oversight provided by the judiciary having a crucial role in this case. Civil rights actions can also serve an important role in deterring possible overreach by states in using their public health powers. On October 22, 2015—exactly one year after departing Sierra Leone—Kaci Hickox lodged a civil rights action against New Jersey Governor Christie and other officials alleging violations of her Constitutional rights, including her Fourteenth Amendment rights. If successful, this case may provide a legal deterrent to the future imposition of mandatory quarantines beyond the scope of the CDC's guidelines.

Legal Solutions to Gaps in Pandemic Preparedness

As the 2013–2016 EVD outbreak demonstrated, despite the existence of strong federal and state public health law powers, differing understandings of state law can derail an effective global and public health response. As the Hickox case demonstrates, interpretations of existing state public health powers can vary greatly from the legal reality once tested by a court. State political leaders must ensure that they understand the extent of their legal powers, and if necessary, revise and clarify state legislation. In addition, state and federal priorities are likely to vary greatly. During the 2013–2016 EVD outbreak, the US federal government's priorities included protecting national health by stopping the outbreak in West Africa; its international legal obligations; and foreign policy considerations. These priorities are unlikely to match states' much narrower priority of protecting the health or addressing the concerns of their citizens. In addition, even these same priorities will have varying policy goals for each state, resulting in vastly different outcomes. An effective domestic legal and public health response requires consistency as well as flexibility. Two possible approaches—one hardline, one collaborative—may provide this: preemption and cooperative agreements.

Preemption

Federal preemption is the invalidation of a state law due to a conflict with a federal law under the Supremacy Clause of the US Constitution. One of the main justifications for preemption is the need for uniformity between federal and state laws.[49] For example, state quarantine laws that govern interstate movement have been preempted insofar as they conflict with federal laws.[50]

Understandably, the use of federal preemption can be controversial. Congress attempts to prevent inadvertent federal preemption of state laws by including anti-preemption clauses in legislation. The Public Health Services Act contains an anti-preemption clause, but is limited in its application. State public health measures—such as mandatory quarantines—above the federal regulation may not be interpreted as in conflict with federal laws, but rather setting a higher standard above the federal minimum. Yet if the state law essentially acts as an obstacle to federal laws, it may conflict and therefore be preempted.[51] It is feasible that given the broader national health security aims of the federal government, the effectiveness of the CDC's federal regulations were undermined by state laws during the US Ebola pandemic response, legitimizing a federal preemption argument. States are, however, unlikely to welcome federal preemption of their pandemic response laws. Furthermore, a hardline approach and legal conflict between states and the federal government may further undermine federal-state cooperation necessary for the US domestic pandemic response.

Cooperation Agreements

Some federations use cooperation agreements in an attempt to preempt the legal and political dynamics that might arise due to threats to public health security, by establishing a framework for clear, fast, and informed decision making during disease outbreaks that may quickly spread nationally.[52] While not a formal delegation of power from the states to the federal government, state and federal governments agree to coordinate and cooperate in their responses to public health crises. Such documents can include an agreement that states defer to the advice of a federal regulatory body—such as the CDC—in scientific or technical matters. It could also include model public health legislation for states to implement at their discretion and subject to their own democratic processes. While this is not a formal delegation of power, and states retain their sovereignty to withdraw from the agreement or parts of the agreement, this nonbinding collaborative approach may provide certainty for matters such as recommended health measures. In exchange, the federal government may provide forms of support to states such as funding or coordination assistance without resorting to legislative emergency powers. While it is unlikely that complete agreement would be reached across all 50 of the US states, given the possibilities of top-down, hard-line options such as preemption available to the federal government, a cooperative agreement would help facilitate the necessary discussion for clearer federal and state laws for US public health preparedness.

Conclusion

The US federal and state legal responses to the 2013–2016 EVD outbreak were substantially varied, and political pressure risked undermining the United States's important role as a leader in strengthening the IHR and global health security. Even where legitimate legal powers existed, the Ebola outbreak served as a sentinel for their potential use to achieve narrow goals, potentially undermining national public health and security. While the spread of Ebola in the United States was limited, in preparation for future infectious disease outbreaks, state and federal government priorities and legal authorities should be aligned for a more coordinated and effective response. Although the federal government may be able to use federal preemption to enforce this, such an approach should be judiciously considered. Alternative models—such as a cooperative agreement or model laws—may provide a solution or, at the very least, facilitate the necessary discussion for clearer and more efficient US public health legal preparedness.

Notes

1. World Health Organization, *Constitution of the World Health Organization*, 45th ed., e-book (Geneva: World Health Organization, 2006), articles 21 and 22, http://www.who.int/governance/eb/who_constitution_en.pdf. Countries may "opt out" of the IHR obligations only in very specific circumstances, set out in World Health Organization, *International Health Regulations 2005*, 2nd ed. (Geneva: World Health Organization, 2008), http://whqlibdoc.who.int/publications/2008/9789241580410

_eng.pdf IHR, articles 59, 61 and 62. The United States was one of only two countries to formally submit any reservations to the IHR. Of particular relevance here, the United States submitted a reservation that its obligations under the IHR are to be interpreted in a "manner consistent with its fundamental principles of federalism," and that where such obligations "come under the legal jurisdiction of the state governments, the [US] Federal Government shall bring such obligations with a favorable recommendation to the notice of the appropriate state authorities"; see World Health Organization, *International Health Regulations 2005*, appendix 2.

2. CDC, "Cases of Ebola Diagnosed in the United States," last updated December 16, 2014, http://www.cdc.gov/vhf/ebola/outbreaks/2014-west-africa/united-states-imported-case.html. This site does not include individuals diagnosed with Ebola overseas but repatriated to the United States for treatment: Samaritan's Purse doctor Kent Brantly and missionary Nancy Writebol, who both survived after evacuation for treatment at Emory University Hospital in Atlanta, Georgia, and US resident Dr. Martin Salia, who died after evacuation for treatment at the Nebraska Medical Center in Omaha, Nebraska.

3. US Constitution, art. 1, sec. 8, cl. 3.

4. Other US constitutional powers—such as the national defense powers—may be used to respond to infectious disease outbreaks in light of the increased securitization of public health threats, whether naturally or intentionally occurring. See, for example, Laura K. Donohue, "Pandemic Disease, Biological Weapons, and War" in *Law And War*, eds. Austin Sarat, Lawrence Douglas, and Martha Merrill Umphrey (Palo Alto: Stanford University Press, 2014).

5. Affected and neighboring countries, in particular Sierra Leone and Liberia, implemented various forms of border closures to strengthen attempts to contain EVD; these measures were permitted by the WHO temporary recommendations. See Umaru Fofana, "Sierra Leone Shuts Borders, Closes Schools to Fight Ebola," Reuters UK, June 11, 2014, http://uk.reuters.com/article/2014/06/11/us-health-ebola-leone-idUKKBN0EM2CG20140611; Charlotte Alter, "Liberia Closes Borders to Curb Ebola Outbreak," *Time*, July 28, 2014, http://time.com/3046012/liberia-border-ebola/; US Overseas Security Advisory Council, "Security Message for U.S. Citizens: Dakar (Senegal), Border Closures due to Ebola Virus Disease," August 25, 2014, https://www.osac.gov/pages/ContentReportDetails.aspx?cid=16206.

6. "Ebola Virus Letter to President Obama," October 8, 2014, http://www.scribd.com/doc/242444231/Ebola-Virus-Letter-to-President-Obama-10-8-2014.

7. Ibid.

8. President Barack Obama, "What You Need to Know about Ebola," White House weekly address, October 18, 2014, https://www.whitehouse.gov/photos-and-video/video/2014/10/18/weekly-address-what-you-need-know-about-ebola.

9. Modeling for a hypothetical novel influenza outbreak in the United States concluded that border closures, even if 99.9% effective, would only delay the disease peak in the United States by six weeks. See Neil M. Ferguson, D. A. Cummings, C. Fraser, J. C. Cajka, P. C. Cooley, D. S. Burke, "Strategies for Mitigating an Influenza Pandemic," *Nature* 442, no. 7101 (July 27, 2006): 449. Similarly, US measures initiated in the 1980s banning the entry of HIV-positive individuals were ineffective, and rather contributed to stigmatization: see Matthew J. DeFazio, "Guarding International Borders Against HIV: A Comparative Study in Futility," *Pace International Law Review* 25 (2013): 89.

10. See, generally, Jack Nicas and Susan Carey, "Travel Ban over Ebola May Bring Other Troubles," *Wall Street Journal*, October 19, 2014, http://www.wsj.com/articles/travel-ban-over-ebola-may-bring-other-troubles-1413748220; Heidi Vogt, "Travel Restrictions Hamper African Medical Staff in Ebola Fight," *Wall Street Journal*, October 24, 2014, http://www.wsj.com/articles/travel-restrictions-hamper-african-medical-staff-in-ebola-fight-1414086147.

11. Ibid.

12. Under the IHR, if a country imposes health measures that significantly interfere with international traffic, it must submit to the WHO its public health rationale and the relevant scientific information for its decision.[1] Without a legitimate public health or scientific basis to travel bans, the United States would have likely breached its obligations under the IHR if travel bans were implemented.

13. Helen Branswell, "Ebola: Canada Suspending Visas for Residents of Outbreak Countries," October 31, 2014, CBC News, http://www.cbc.ca/news/politics/ebola-canada-suspending-visas-for-residents-of-outbreak-countries-1.2820090.

14. Incorporation of a sanctions regime into the IHR is a long-standing issue. In response to the 2013–2016 Ebola outbreak, in October 2015 the WHO Director-General Margaret Chan called for accountability mechanisms to be included in the IHR. See Lisa De Bode, "WHO Wants Sanctions Against Countries for Mishandling Epidemic," October 22, 2015, Al Jazeera America, http://america.aljazeera.com/articles/2015/10/22/health-sanctions-against-countries-misguided.html.

15. Clive M. Brown, Aaron E. Aranas, Gabrielle A. Benenson, Gary Brunette, Marty Cetron, Tai-Ho Chen, et al., "Airport Exit and Entry Screening for Ebola-August-November 10, 2014," *Morbidity and Mortality Weekly Report* 63, no. 49 (2014): 1163–67.

16. Ibid.

17. IHR, art. 23, sec. 1a.

18. Liberian government authorities, including President Ellen Johnson Sirleaf, accused Mr. Duncan of lying about his contact with possible EVD on his airport

departure questionnaire and stated that they intended to prosecute him on his return. Mr. Duncan was unable to personally respond to the accusations and passed away on October 8, 2014 from EVD. See Norimitsu Onishi and Marc Santora, "Ebola Patient in Dallas Lied on Screening Form, Liberian Airport Official Says," *The New York Times,* October 2, 2014, http://www.nytimes.com/2014/10/03/world/africa/dallas-ebola-patient-thomas-duncan-airport-screening.html.

19. See Craig Spencer, "Having and Fighting Ebola—Public Health Lessons from a Clinician Turned Patient," *New England Journal of Medicine* 372 (2015): 1089–91.

20. The two other EVD cases diagnosed within the United States were not subject to border screening, as both were nurses who contracted the illness within the United States while treating Mr. Duncan.

21. See, for example, "Effort to Prevent Panic over Ebola Went Too Far," *Los Angeles Times,* editorial, October 8, 2014, http://www.latimes.com/opinion/editorials/la-ed-ebola-obama-cdc-precautions-20141009-story.html.

22. Lawrence O. Gostin, *Public Health Law: Power, Duty, Restraint,* 2nd ed. (California: University of California Press, 2008), 461.

23. David L. Heymann, ed., *Control of Communicable Diseases Manual,* 18th ed. (Washington, DC: American Public Health Association, 2004), 621, as cited in Gostin, *Public Health Law: Power, Duty, Restraint.*

24. Ibid., 617–19.

25. See for example, the Australian Commonwealth of Australia Constitution Act, 1900 (Imp), sec. 51 (ix), and the Canadian Constitution Act, 1867, sec. 91 (11).

26. Public Health Service Act 42, US Code 264, sec. 361.

27. 42 CFR part 71.

28. 42 CFR part 70.

29. Executive order no. 13295, sec. 5, April 4, 2003, 68 F.R. 17255, amended by executive order no. 13375, sec. 1, April 1, 2005, 70 F.R. 17255, and by executive order no. 13674, sec. 1, July 31, 2014, 79 F.R. 45671.

30. "In general, CDC defers to state and local health authorities in their primary use of their own separate quarantine powers. Based upon long experience and collaborative working relationships with our state and local partners, CDC continues to anticipate the need to use this federal authority to quarantine an exposed person only in rare situations, such as events at ports of entry or in similar time-sensitive settings"; see CDC, "Questions and Answers on the Executive Order Adding Potentially Pandemic Influenza Viruses to the List of Quarantinable Diseases," last updated October 22, 2015, http://www.cdc.gov/quarantine/qa-executive-order-pandemic-list-quarantinable-diseases.html.

31. This position was unanimously confirmed by the Supreme Court nearly 200 years ago in *Gibbons v Ogden,* 22 US 9 Wheat. 11 (1824), in which Chief Justice John Marshall held that enacting quarantine laws are among the powers reserved for the states.

32. Lawrence Gostin, "The Future of Public Health Law," *American Journal of Law and Medicine* 12 (1987): 461–490.

33. Reasonableness as a determinative factor in a legitimate quarantine was articulated in *Jew Ho v Williamson,* 103 F. 10 N.D. Cal. (1900), rejecting a quarantine that was "unreasonable, unjust, and oppressive and therefore contrary to the laws limiting the police powers of the state" at [26] and subsequently reinforced by *Jacobson v Massachusetts* 197 US 11 (1905).

34. CDC, "CDC Interim Guidance for Monitoring and Movement of People Exposed to Ebola Virus," last updated February 19, 2016, http://www.cdc.gov/vhf/ebola/exposure/monitoring-and-movement-of-persons-with-exposure.html.

35. For a detailed analysis of the different responses to returned travelers between states, see John D. Kraemer, Mark J. Siedner, and Michael A. Stoto, "Analyzing Variability in Ebola-Related Controls Applied to Returned Travelers in the United States," *Health Security* 15 (2015): 295–306.

36. California Department of Public Health, "State Health Officer Issues Risk-Based Quarantine Order to Provide Consistent Guidelines for Counties," October 29, 2014, http://www.cdph.ca.gov/Pages/NR14-089.aspx.

37. Governor Dannel P. Malloy, "Gov. Malloy outlines state's policies for monitoring travelers from Guinea, Liberia, and Sierra Leone," October 27, 2014, http://portal.ct.gov/Gov-Malloy-Outlines-State-s-Policies-for-Monitoring-Travelers-from-Guinea-Liberia-and-Sierra-Leone/.

38. Office of the governor of Florida, "Gov. Scott Issues Executive Order Requiring Mandatory Health Monitoring for Anyone Returning from Ebola-Affected Areas," October 25, 2014, http://www.flgov.com/2014/10/25/gov-scott-issues-executive-order-requiring-mandatory-health-monitoring-for-anyone-returning-from-ebola-affected-areas-2/.

39. Office of the governor of the State of Georgia, "Deal Issues New Policy for Travelers from Ebola-Affected Countries," October 27, 2014, http://gov.georgia.gov/press-releases/2014-10-27/deal-issues-new-policy-travelers-ebola-affected-countries.

40. Illinois Department of Public Health, "Illinois Department of Public Health Issues Ebola Safety Guidance," October 27, 2014, http://www.idph.state.il.us/public/press14/10.27.14_IDPH_Issues_Ebola_Safety_Guidance.htm.

41. Described as "voluntary, in-home quarantine," but if an individual refuses, Maine would "take additional measures and pursue appropriate authority to ensure

they make no public contact"; Commissioner Mary Mayhew, "Commissioner Discusses Ebola Protocols," October 28, 2014, http://www.maine.gov/tools/whatsnew/index.php?topic=DHS+Press+Releases&id=630405&v=article.

42. Scott Dance, "Md. to impose Home Quarantine, Transit Limits on Some Travelers from Ebola-Stricken Countries," *Baltimore Sun,* October 27, 2014, http://www.baltimoresun.com/health/bs-hs-maryland-ebola-quarantine-20141027-story.html.

43. Justin Worland, "Christie and Cuomo Announce Mandatory Ebola Quarantine," *TIME,* October 25, 2014, http://time.com/3537755/ebola-new-york-new-jersey/.

44. Ibid.

45. Ibid.

46. Plaintiff's submissions, *Hickox v Christie et al.* (2:15-cv-07647), New Jersey District Court, filed October 22, 2015.

47. 22 M.R.S. § 811(3) (2014).

48. *Maine v Hickox* (CV-2014–36), Maine District Court, October 30, 2015.

49. Mary J. Davis, "Unmasking the Presumption in Favor of Preemption," *South Carolina Law Review* 53, no. 967 (2002): 1016.

50. *Morgan's Steamship Co. v Board of Health of the State of Louisiana,* 118 US 455 (1886), 464: "For while it may be a police power in the sense that all provisions for health, comfort, and security of the citizens are police regulations, and an exercise of the police power, even where such powers are so exercised as to come within the domain of federal authority as defined in the constitution, the latter must prevail." Similarly, in the seminal case *Jacobson v Massachusetts,* 197 US 11, 25 (1905), the court noted at [25] that "[a] local enactment of regulation, even if based on the acknowledged police powers of a state, must always yield in case of conflict with the exercise by the general government of any power it possesses under the Constitution, or with any right which that instrument gives or secures."

51. A full discussion of obstacle preemption is beyond the scope of this chapter. However, see, for example, *Crosby v. National Foreign Trade Council,* 530 US 363, 373–74 (2000).

52. See, for example, the Coalition of Australian Governments "National Health Security Agreement," 2008.

IV Mainstream and Social Media Response

10 Talking about Ebola: Medical Journalism in an Age of Social Media

Cyril Ibe

Ebola Appears in the United States

The 2013–2016 outbreak of Ebola virus disease (EVD) first hit remote parts of Guinea in March 2013. The virus then crossed unannounced to neighboring Liberia in the summer before moving on to Sierra Leone, unleashing untold human misery and wreaking extraordinary public health havoc in these impoverished West African countries.

Liberia was the hardest hit, with daily death tolls in the tens. For some time, the outbreak failed to capture news headlines in the United States—at least not until a seminal Ebola-related incident in Dallas, Texas. By the end of September 2014, this unprecedented event, linked to importation of the virus from Liberia, dramatically changed all that, sending the developed nation on an emotionally charged Ebola alert.

As the largest Ebola outbreak ever recorded percolated, resulting in thousands of deaths in Liberia alone by mid-September 2014, it began to rapidly dominate international news headlines and conversations on social media across the globe. "On Twitter, a whopping 10.5 million tweets mentioning the word 'Ebola' were sent between Sept. 16 and Oct. 6 from 170 countries around the world," wrote technology reporter Victor Luckerson on Time.com on October 7, 2014.[1]

October 7 was one week after Thomas Eric Duncan, a 42-year-old Liberian national who had traveled from his country to reunite with his fiancé in Dallas, was confirmed to have EVD at Texas Health Presbyterian Hospital in Dallas. This marked the first time an Ebola infection had been diagnosed on American soil, and, overnight, news of the West African immigrant's diagnosis elevated Ebola to a water-cooler-and-dinner-table conversation topic and lit up the Twittersphere in record numbers.

"On the night of Oct. 1, Twitter users were firing off missives about Ebola at the rate of more than 6,000 per minute, up from about 100 per minute before Sept. 30," Luckerson reported, citing "exclusive Twitter data" Time magazine had obtained.[2]

"The country where Ebola dominates conversation most is Liberia, where the virus has already claimed more than 2,000 lives. In terms of sheer volume, though, most Ebola tweets are sent from the United States," Time.com reported.[3] Veteran Dallas television medical reporter Janet St. James was among those jamming up Twitter to bring the far-away Ebola story out of West Africa home to a frightened American audience.

On September 30, St. James scooped all her news competitors—in print, broadcast, and online media—by breaking the news that Duncan was being tested for Ebola at the Dallas hospital exclusively on Twitter. The next day, October 1, she outwitted them again on Twitter with Duncan's positive Ebola diagnosis.

"Twitter is much more immediate than the news [on television] is," explained St. James in a phone interview. "I didn't have to wait for there to be a newscast. I could break it on Twitter and I knew that people would get the news much faster. Once I chose to break it [on Twitter], I knew that it could go multiple other places and people could share it."[4]

The WFAA-TV news reporter had been on the medical beat for more than 15 years in the Dallas-Fort Worth area. St. James is one of a rapidly growing number of medical reporters who welcome social media as both tools and allies on their beats in the convergent journalism era of the twenty-first century.

St. James deliberately circumvented her traditional medium of television in favor of Twitter—with its unique power to connect its users instantaneously with a global audience of followers. "I knew that I was going to break [the Ebola news] exactly the way I wanted it phrased" more or less without a gatekeeper, she said.[5] "I broke the story in the evening probably at 8:30 or 9. I was at home so I could break this news from the comfort of my kitchen," St. James added.[6] After St. James broke the Duncan story, Duncan's positive EVD diagnosis shook not just the Dallas hospital and dwellers of the Dallas-Fort Worth metropolis, but also Americans of all political and social persuasions. The US Centers for Disease Control and Prevention (CDC), public health departments, and public and private hospitals around the country were equally on high alert. With the explosion of Ebola messages on Twitter and Facebook and American television networks including CNN dubbing Ebola "the ISIS of biological agents,"[7] the United States was figuratively on an Ebola lockdown.

Duncan never left the Dallas hospital. He died there on October 8, 2014, just days after his diagnosis and short-lived treatment. Days later, two nurses who cared for him in the hospital, Nina Pham and Amber Vinson, tested positive for the Ebola virus, further heightening the public health urgency of eliminating further transmission in America.

Ebola Treatments at Emory University Hospital

Pham and Vinson were the first individuals to become infected with the Ebola virus within the borders of the United States. Pham was admitted and treated at the National Institutes of Health Clinical Center in Bethesda, Maryland, from which she was discharged on October 16. Admitted at Emory University Hospital in Atlanta, Vinson was another high-profile patient because of her travel to the Cleveland area to visit family and shop for a bridal gown, despite her exposure to Ebola. She was discharged from Emory on October 28, the fourth patient treated there.

Dr. Kent Brantly and Nancy Writebol, who were the first EVD patients to be treated in the United States, had been admitted at Emory in early August 2014. They became infected with the Ebola virus during their stints as humanitarian aid workers in Liberia. Writebol was discharged August 19, and Brantly followed on August 21. A third patient who declined to be identified publicly was admitted at Emory on September 9 and discharged on October 19. All four patients were treated in Emory's Serious Communicable Disease Unit, which was established 12 years ago jointly with the CDC to care for CDC scientists and others who get exposed to infectious diseases during travels abroad.

If social media had become helpful tools for reporter St. James, their benefits were a mixed bag for Emory. Despite the successful EVD treatments, Emory was not unscathed by innuendos that were rampant on Twitter and other social media as patients were admitted to the specially equipped unit at Emory, said university spokesman Vince Dollard in a phone interview.[8] Consider this tweet on October 20, 2014 from @moneyries, following the discharge of an unidentified Ebola patient from Emory the day before: "Emory University had an Ebola patient this whole time and nobody knew it. Well done."[9] The tweet implied a cover-up by hospital officials.

"Social media was vitriolic, but the tide overwhelmingly turned and our supporters began to weigh in. The number of supporters outweighed our detractors," Dollard said in the interview.[10]

"In the first few days of the Ebola issue—July 31 through the first week of August 2014—I read comments such as: 'People who go to Africa deserve to die,' 'People who care for those people are crazy,' comments along those lines, including opinions such as Ebola patients shouldn't be allowed back in this country," added Nancy Seideman, Emory University's senior spokesman.[11]

"We were able to shift the national social media conversation with Susan M. Grant's *Washington Post* op-ed that ended with the line: 'We can fear, or we can care.'[12] This op-ed was picked up widely by mainstream and social media, and as a result of this op-ed—and the accurate information consistently provided by Emory, the CDC, and other organizations—and media coverage—the social media negativity trended way down, and remained down," said Seideman.[13]

Under Intense Fire, CDC Fights Back with Social Media

For its part, the CDC also faced an unrelenting social media barrage, from both a highly anxious American public and elected US officials, for its handling of the Ebola outbreak (how the CDC found itself in this situation is covered by Marjorie Kruvand in chapter 11). Some of the biting criticism was directed at what some considered the agency's lack of an emergency protocol on how to not only protect health care workers like Pham and Vinson, but also how to stop the Ebola virus at US borders and entry points.

Wall Street Journal editorial page writer Sohrab Ahmari slammed both the CDC and the World Health Organization for "shameful, incompetent, slow" bureaucracy in handling the EVD outbreak.[14]

A scathing October 16, 2014 *Newsday* editorial titled "CDC must get its act together on Ebola" blasted the head of the CDC.[15]

"Dr. Thomas Frieden, who runs the U.S. Centers for Disease Control and Prevention, learned Thursday what happens when a crucial American health sentry is caught snoozing during an invasion," it read.[16]

The editorial continued: "The agency charged with keeping America safe from life-threatening illnesses was forced to face hard questions from a congressional subcommittee—and to admit that it didn't know exactly how two nurses contracted the Ebola virus from patient Thomas Eric Duncan in Dallas."[17]

As the criticisms flew like arrows from several angles—from press and public attacks to heated congressional hearings—the CDC also took to social media to defend itself.

"CDC joined the social conversation where and when it was occurring," explained Jessica Schindelar, a health communication specialist in the CDC's digital media branch. The CDC disseminated more than 200 messages across social media platforms during the first week of August 2014, as the Ebola outbreak was picking up steam in US media.[18]

"People are getting more information from different sources than ever before, especially nontraditional ones like social media," Schindelar continued. "This provides an opportunity for trusted sources like us at CDC to share reliable, scientifically accurate information with multiple audiences, including the general public, via their preferred channel."[19]

From monitoring trends on social media regarding Ebola to identifying rumors and misconceptions to filling information gaps, Schindelar said CDC's social media use was as steady as it was unabashed.[20]

The Donald Trump Factor

Tweets[21] by business and real estate magnate Donald Trump about Ebola were among some of the boldest and most controversial public criticisms. "I have been saying for weeks for President Obama to stop the flights from West Africa. So simple, but he refused. A TOTAL incompetent!" Trump tweeted from @realDonaldTrump on October 23, 2014, to at least two million followers.

While Trump's numerous Ebola tweets fanned panic and fear in Americans, the CDC's communication on social media was aimed both to counter and to clarify.

"During the height of the Ebola outbreak, one of the biggest misconceptions we identified and clarified [on] social media was about why health care workers wear so much personal protective equipment if Ebola is not airborne. It is because CDC recommends health care workers wear protective gear due to the possibility of large amounts of blood, other body fluids, vomit, or feces present in the environment," Schindelar said.[22]

"A game changer" was Schindelar's characterization of the CDC's health and crisis communication in highlighting the work its experts, health care professionals, and global public health partners "do every day to prevent and control the spread of disease around the world." The benefits of communicating via social media warrant their continued deployment in public health communication. "An outpouring of appreciation and support [of the experts, health care professionals, and global public health partners] continues to grow out of the sharing of their experiences on social media," Schindelar explained.[23]

Louisiana's Unusual Step to Keep Ebola at Bay

If the CDC was fighting to maintain its image and credibility, Louisiana officials were more bent on keeping Ebola at bay from their state. By late October 2014, they adopted a unique, if contentious, prescription to prevent "unnecessary exposure of Ebola to the general public." Kathy Kliebert, secretary of the Department of Health and Hospitals (DHH) in Louisiana, and Kevin Davis, the director of the Governor's Office of Homeland Security and Emergency Preparedness,[24] jointly requested that all individuals who had traveled to Ebola-affected countries in West Africa voluntarily quarantine themselves for 21 days following their travel history with or without symptoms. Furthermore, they disinvited several experts among about 4,000 people preparing to attend the 63rd annual meeting of the American Society of Tropical Medicine and Hygiene slated for November 2–6, 2014, in New Orleans, Louisiana. Nevertheless, the officials admitted this was more a precautionary measure than one based on science.

"Individuals who have traveled to and returned from the countries of Sierra Leone, Liberia, or Guinea in the past 21 days, or have had contact with a known [Ebola] patient in that time period, should not travel to New Orleans to attend the conference. Given that conference participants with a travel and exposure history for [Ebola] are recommended not to participate in large group settings (such as this conference) or to utilize public transport, we see no utility in you traveling to New Orleans to simply be confined to your room," stated the email signed by Kliebert and Davis.[25] Government officials required ASTMH to pass on the email message.

"We certainly respected the work of the conference attendees, but our big obligation was to the public health of all Louisiana residents and the conference attendees as well. Certainly, in the abundance of caution, we felt it was best to issue the public health advisory for the conference attendees planning to visit New Orleans," Kliebert explained in a phone interview.[26]

Like health reporters breaking news on Twitter and holding conversations with their audience on Facebook, Louisiana public health officials engaged with their constituents via Twitter and Facebook primarily, providing them information for re-tweeting or posting on Facebook walls.

"We know that social media is the place where individuals go to share their frustration, their fears, they ask questions of one another. So it's critical that, as a public health entity, we share accurate, timely information to help individuals feel reassured so that they know what the state is doing to help protect their health and safety," said Olivia Watkins Hwang, director of media and communications for Louisiana's Department of Health and Hospitals.[27]

"The strategy for social media isn't very different [from] a general strategy for crisis communication. You want to be first, you want to be accurate, you want to be timely, and you want to give people something that makes them feel reassured, that makes them feel empowered. So information about things they can do, or steps they can take, or things they can be aware of is always critical to emergency-response communication," Hwang said. "That was part of our strategy with Ebola."[28]

Summit County's Local Response to Ebola

A brief visit to her family in Summit County in Ohio by Amber Vinson, the second Dallas nurse infected with Ebola, thrust public health officials there into crisis communication high gear. A local, national, and international news spotlight focused on Summit County, as social media and the 24-hour news cycle became a dual challenge for health officials.

"We, in the very early hours of this incident, started monitoring social media. ... We are a small health department. ... So this was an overwhelming presence, the whole Ebola situation," said public health information officer Marlene Martin in a phone interview. "So very early on, our emergency operation center was opened in our county. We also had someone stationed in there that was monitoring social media for us as well."[29]

Rather than chase and respond to every social media rumor or misconception on the Ebola connection to Summit County, even from talking heads on national television, officials were determined to counter with expert information on the virus in an effort to calm the flared-up nerves of their constituents.

"Again, we felt it [was] very important to get out the information, the facts [about Ebola], and so we didn't take a lot of time to respond to people who were saying strange things and mean things on social media," Martin said. "We were just reinforcing that we were putting out the truth: This is how it is contracted, these are the symptoms."[30]

Television talking heads and "so-called experts" had it wrong most of the time about how Ebola is transmitted, according to Dr. Marguerite Erme, medical director of Summit County (Ohio). "Dealing with some of the information that came out on the news media, on what people's opinions [were] and having to counteract that with science, was a little challenging. The people who were talking the most about this on the news were not the people who know the most but the people who are the most recognized, and they weren't always the best educated [on Ebola]," she said.[31]

Ebola Studies and Social Media Power

If the 2014 Ebola outbreak in an age of social media posed communication challenges to public health officials like those in Summit County, it offered scholars opportunities for research on how people were seeking information about the disease, tracking its spread, and voicing concern over it among various users and populations.

One study used trend data from Twitter and Google searches in late September 2014 when the first Ebola diagnosis in the United States was confirmed to draw conclusions that television news clips drove Americans into panic and sent them querying "Ebola symptoms" and whether or not they were free of Ebola.[32] The study analyzed Ebola-related news video broadcast on Fox News and MSNBC networks to assess how they spurred tweets and Google searches on Ebola.

"It appears that basically every news video that was aired—Ebola-related news video—inspired thousands of tweets and internet searches related to Ebola," explained study co-author Sherry Towers of Arizona State University's Simon A. Levin Mathematical, Computational, and Modeling Sciences Center in a phone interview.[33]

"And the Internet searches ranged from searches that perhaps reflect simple curiosity, like people searching for information on Ebola symptoms to people doing Google searches relating to such terms as 'Do I have Ebola,' which reflects something more than simple curiosity. It appears that the news media [were] actually—you can call it somewhat contagious in inspiring people to do Ebola-related tweets or internet searches" during the period that was studied.

Is Social Media Good for Health Reporting?

As much as social media helps the medical reporter break news scoops and engage in ongoing conversations with his or her audience members, some lament that it robs health reporting of the necessary depth and context often associated with it.

"In fact, having had a long background in traditional media, I find that the growing reliance on social media feeds the negative trend of minimizing detail and context in reporting," said Earle Holland, a former newspaper and science reporter for more than 35 years. "The constraints of social media, coupled with the lack of editorial oversight in almost all cases, [are] a major limiting factor in providing comprehensive and complex reporting."[34]

Emory University's Seideman acknowledged that social media often provides a forum where users can counter misinformation by offering "accurate" information and even drum up empathy, as was eventually the case with Ebola patients. "Social media can be wonderful at self-correcting when you let issues play out."[35]

As for medical reporters who use social media, Seideman offered a caveat. "As always with social media, traditional media representatives need to check the accuracy of all information shared and consider the source of all information, particularly when dealing with medical issues," she said.[36]

Holland concurred and also elaborated.

"Medical journalism has a great responsibility to its readers, given that the news it provides directly affects people's well-being. Patients, and their families and friends, deserve to receive relevant medical information in the proper context. Social media inherently can't do that since it is more oriented towards speed than completeness, and context—how the story fits into a larger perspective—is almost always missing," he said.[37]

Any Social Media Lessons Learned?

WFAA-TV's Janet St. James comfortably and conveniently broke her Ebola stories in Dallas, Texas, using Twitter and Facebook, which she considers important reporting tools in modern journalism. For that, she has nothing but counsel for both budding and seasoned journalists in the use of social media.

"The lesson for me is that you can shape the message and shape it responsibly on social media," she said. "It doesn't always have to be about rumors and innuendos. Social media can also be about facts, not fear.[38]

"I think [journalists] should become comfortable with [social media]. Most of us didn't grow up using social media, so I think they should become comfortable with it, how to phrase it and how to use in an accurate and timely manner. I think that's critical for all reporters."[39]

Notes

1. Victor Luckerson, "Watch How Ebola Exploded in America," *Time*, http://time.com/3478452/ebola-twitter/.

2. Ibid.

3. Ibid.

4. Janet St. James (medical journalist) in discussion with the author, May 2015.

5. Ibid.

6. Ibid.

7. "CNN concedes Ebola is not in fact 'ISIS of biological agents,'" CNN, YouTube video, October 6, 2014, https://www.YouTube.com/watch?v=XrovH26DlbA.

8. Vince Dollard, e-mail message to author, July 7, 2015.

9. Brian Reis, Twitter post, January 14, 2016, 5:27 p.m., https://twitter.com/search?q=%40moneyries%20ebola&src=typd.

10. Vince Dollard, e-mail message to author, July 7, 2015.

11. Nancy Seideman, e-mail message to author, July 9, 2015.

12. Susan Grant, "I'm the head nurse at Emory. This is why we wanted to bring the Ebola patients to the U.S.," Post Everything (blog), *Washington Post,* August 6, 2014, https://www.washingtonpost.com/posteverything/wp/2014/08/06/im-the-head-nurse-at-emory-this-is-why-we-wanted-to-bring-the-ebola-patients-to-the-u-s/.

13. Nancy Seideman, e-mail message to author, July 9, 2015.

14. Sohrab Ahmari, "Opinion: Ebola Takes Down the Bureaucracies" (video), *Wall Street Journal,* October 16, 2014, http://www.wsj.com/video/opinion-ebola-takes-down-the-bureaucracies/CC42D6F1-A2E9-46ED-92E2-5061DADA8AE8.html.

15. "Editorial: CDC Must Get Its Act Together on Ebola," Newsday.com, October 16, 2014, http://www.newsday.com/opinion/cdc-must-get-its-act-together-on-ebola-editorial-1.9513154.

16. Ibid.

17. Ibid.

18. Jessica Schindelar, e-mail message to author, June 26, 2015.

19. Ibid.

20. Ibid.

21. Donald Trump, Twitter post, October 23, 2014, https://twitter.com/realDonaldTrump.

22. Jessica Schindelar, e-mail message to author, June 26, 2015.

23. Ibid.

24. Kathy Kliebert and Kevin Davis, "Notice to Travelers," press release, Baton Rouge, Louisiana, 2014.

25. Erica Check Hayden, "Protest Sparked as Louisiana Seeks to Ban Doctors Returned from West Africa," *Nature Magazine,* October 30, 2014, http://www.scientificamerican.com/article/protest-sparked-as-louisiana-seeks-to-ban-doctors-returned-from-west-africa/.

26. Kathy Kliebert (secretary of health) in discussion with author, June 2015.

27. Olivia Watkins Hwang (public health department spokeswoman) in discussion with author, June 2015.

28. Ibid.

29. Marlene Martin (public health department spokeswoman) in discussion with author, May 2015.

30. Ibid.

31. Marguerite Erme (county public health medical director) in discussion with author, May 2015.

32. Sherry Towers, Shehzad Afzal, Gilbert Bernal, Nadya Bliss, Shala Brown, Baltazar Espinoza, et al., "Mass Media and the Contagion of Fear: The Case of Ebola in America," *PLoS One* 10, no. 6 (2015), doi: http://dx.doi.org/10.1371/journal.pone.0129179.

33. Sherry Towers (statistician, modeler) in discussion with author, July 2015.

34. Earle Holland, e-mail message to author, June 30, 2015.

35. Nancy Seideman, e-mail message to author, July 9, 2015.

36. Ibid.

37. Earle Holland, e-mail message to author, June 30, 2015.

38. Janet St. James (medical journalist) in discussion with the author, May 2015.

39. Ibid.

11 Risk Watch: Media Coverage of Ebola in the Digital Communication Era

Cristine Russell

On March 23, 2014, the World Health Organization posted a report on its website of a surprising outbreak of Ebola virus disease (EVD) in the West African nation of Guinea,[1] marking the first time it had appeared in this part of the continent. At that time, at least 29 had died and 49 people had been infected with a highly lethal species of the virus known to kill up to 90 percent of its victims. The global news media paid scant attention.

The international media wake-up call came four months later, with back-to-back events that warned the world this fast-moving EVD epidemic was already the worst in history.[2] By then, the disease had already struck 1,600 people and claimed 880 lives in Guinea and the neighboring countries of Liberia and Sierra Leone.[3]

Alarm one: On August 2, 2014, Ebola arrived in the United States when a physician who contracted the disease while treating patients in Liberia was airlifted 4,750 miles to Emory University Hospital in Atlanta, Georgia. Dr. Kent Brantly[4] underwent intensive care there in a medical isolation unit designed to handle hazardous infectious diseases like Ebola. This frightening disease now had an American face, and the US and international news media stepped up coverage.

Alarm two: On August 8, 2014, World Health Organization (WHO) Director-General Margaret Chan[5] garnered global headlines when she officially declared the Ebola epidemic a public health emergency of international concern. An emergency committee had unanimously advised her to do so, warning that the EVD outbreak constituted such an "extraordinary event" that "a coordinated international response is deemed essential to stop and reverse the international spread of Ebola."[6]

Alarm three: On September 30, 2014, EVD was diagnosed for the first time on American soil. A Liberian traveler, later identified as Thomas Eric

Duncan, flew commercially to visit family in Dallas, Texas. When he fell ill four days later, Duncan sought emergency care at Texas Health Presbyterian Hospital but was mistakenly diagnosed with a sinus infection.[7] Duncan returned to his family's apartment in a densely populated part of Dallas that was home to many African immigrants. When his condition worsened, he was taken by ambulance to the hospital's isolation unit for round-the-clock care and was finally diagnosed with EVD. While medical missionary Brantly survived, Duncan died on October 8, 2014.[8]

Despite the tragic Ebola epidemic then unfolding in West Africa—with 121 deaths in a single day in Sierra Leone alone[9]—the Texas case attracted massive American and global media attention. "I think unfortunately, in the Western media, there are first-world diseases and third-world diseases, and the attention devoted to the latter depends on the threat they pose to us, not on a universal measure of human suffering," said one media commentator.[10]

For an unprepared American and European public with limited knowledge of EVD, buzzwords such as infectious, exotic, lethal, epidemic, and quarantine naturally provoked fear that this deadly disease could spread widely abroad despite authorities' assurances that stronger public health systems and advanced medical care minimized chances of an Ebola outbreak outside of the African continent.

Flawed media coverage of the epidemic raised several red flags described below, signaling failures to communicate with the public, both inside and outside of Africa, in a responsible and timely manner.

• *Gross mismatch between the magnitude of the West African Ebola epidemic and media coverage.* Western news outlets' coverage of the disastrous human and societal tragedy unfolding in Guinea, Liberia, and Sierra Leone was generally too little and too late. When foreign media outlets sent reporters to these countries, they often focused on foreign medical workers or medical resources from their own country. Images of dead bodies in the streets and medical workers in hazmat suits dehumanized the tragic situation and failed to connect the dots between EVD and the underlying poverty, poor hygiene, and precarious health and political systems in Western Africa.

• *Parochial performance by many mainstream media outlets.* A few imported EVD cases in the United States and Europe received a vastly disproportionate amount of coverage and commentary. Sharp financial cutbacks in specialty beat reporters in areas such as science, medicine, and health, as well as in foreign correspondents, also meant that American print and electronic coverage often lacked in-depth knowledge and perspective. The news media have been democratized and globalized, turned upside down by the emergence of the Internet as a 24/7 source of often unverified information.

• *Rumors, misinformation, and fear spread by social media and cable television news channels.* A Twitter storm and political grandstanding by "talking heads" created controversy, confusion, and knee-jerk reactions in terms of quarantine or travel restrictions. A *Washington Post*-ABC News poll[11] found two-thirds of the American public feared a widespread outbreak of EVD; it was dubbed "the next American panic—an anthrax or SARS [severe acute respiratory syndrome] for the social-media age."[12] A New Jersey survey[13] also suggested that those who followed the EVD story most closely had the least accurate information about the disease, seeing it as more contagious than it actually is.

• *Blame the messenger?* While many news outlets and social media certainly deserve criticism for hyperbolic coverage, there is plenty of blame to go around. Other key stakeholders in the global health communication chain failed to provide clear, coordinated, timely, and useful information to the news media and the public. The WHO came under strong criticism for failing to respond more swiftly to the epidemic's early warning signs; its leadership—and that of other agencies—also failed mass communication 101, with overcharged language such as "catastrophe" fueling overblown media coverage. Political leaders making ill-considered comments often sought media attention.

• *Failure of risk communication.* Communicating the risks of Ebola transmission—particularly who was at greatest risk, how, when, and where—was indeed a major challenge. Risk communication messages from public health officials and the news media needed to be better tailored to differing global audiences. Clearly, many West Africans faced enormous personal risk of contracting Ebola, and their countries' weak health systems meant patients there initially received poor to little care. Health workers and foreign journalists in West Africa who wore protective gear greatly reduced their personal risk of contracting Ebola. Under most circumstances, American and global publics were at virtually no personal risk of contracting Ebola.

The Media Response

Many of the communication problems posed by the EVD epidemic are not new. Age-old infectious disease scourges such as cholera, measles, or tuberculosis attract little fanfare, despite their deadly toll. Novel lethal diseases such as SARS and Middle East respiratory syndrome, or MERS, garner headlines when infected travelers carry diseases into areas not expecting an exotic microbial adversary. Medical teams, public health officials, policy makers, politicians, airline executives, and members of the news media at the local, national, and global level seem to play catch-up with each novel public health emergency.

First detected in 1976[14] in remote areas of Central Africa, Ebola emerged as a ferocious infectious foe that killed more than half of its victims (and fueled frightening nonfiction books such as the 1994 bestseller *The Hot Zone*,[15] as well as dramatic novels and films). The 1976 outbreaks in Zaire (then Democratic Republic of the Congo) and neighboring Sudan claimed 431 lives.[16] Sporadic outbreaks over the years have been localized and contained.

The 2013–2016 EVD epidemic was historic in its magnitude and in its location, appearing for the first time in West Africa and moving into urban as well as rural locations. It was initially not recognized locally, and even after Ebola was detected, the global public health community and the news media were slow to wake up to this fast-moving epidemic.

"When you look at the evolution of the crisis, the international community really woke up when the disease got to America and Europe. And yet we should have known that in this interconnected world it was only a matter of time," said former United Nations Secretary-General Kofi Annan,[17] who told the BBC that he was "bitterly disappointed" by the slow response in richer countries.

"The task of covering Ebola is a tricky one for the media. Too much coverage, and we look like we're being exploitative with scare tactics. Too little coverage, and we get blamed for not enlightening our audience of its scope," noted broadcasting consultant Ken White[18] on the respected Poynter Institute global journalism website.

While the term "news media" is often used as if a singular entity, the term is of course pluralistic, reflecting a diversity of outlets whose coverage of the outbreak has ranged from outstanding to abominable.

At one end of the spectrum, the *New York Times'* exceptional coverage of the EVD outbreak within West Africa earned the newspaper two 2015 Pulitzer Prizes, one for International Reporting and another for Feature Photography. The *Times'* website[19] noted that the newspaper "mobilized dozens of reporters, photographers, video journalists and others over the last year, producing more than 400 articles, including about 50 front-page articles from inside the Ebola-afflicted countries." The sheer amount and quality of the *Times'* coverage demonstrated the opportunities available when a prominent news outlet makes an institutional commitment to use its print and multimedia resources to tackle a challenging, complex story like the EVD outbreak.

When news outlets did have specialty health and science reporters, the coverage generally got high marks. "For the most part, the reporting on medical aspects of the disease has been straightforward and responsible, with many stories emphasizing the relatively low risks of infection," wrote *Washington Post* media reporter Paul Farhi.[20]

A *Columbia Journalism Review* (CJR) article[21] by this author reached a similar conclusion: "The most effective Ebola media coverage thus far has been due in part to the steady hands of experienced—and highly credible—federal medical leaders as well as health and science specialty beat reporters on news teams at major print, radio, and television outlets."

American cable news networks with global reach have rightfully come under considerable criticism for their misleading, fear-mongering Ebola coverage. In their fierce round-the-clock competition for viewers, CNN and Fox News performed especially poorly during live coverage of the first Dallas EVD case, which involved medical mishaps as well as the subsequent infections of two hospital nurses who cared for the Liberian patient.

For example, Fox News Sunday anchor Chris Wallace[22] pushed the federal government's senior infectious disease official Dr. Anthony Fauci, head of the National Institute of Allergy and Infectious Diseases (NIAID), to comment on some farfetched hypotheticals, including whether immigrants on the US southern border were bringing Ebola into the country or whether the Ebola virus would make a good bioterrorism weapon. Fauci quickly dismissed Wallace's scenarios.

Cable network CNN linked two frightening terrors in a shrill on-screen headline: "Ebola: 'The ISIS of Biological Agents?'"[23] CNN anchor Ashleigh

Banfield even suggested ISIS could "send a few of its suicide killers into an Ebola-affected zone and then get them onto mass transit."

"I wish everybody could take a deep breath and take a break from trying to pull viewers in by scaring them," said PBS NewsHour science correspondent Miles O'Brien.[24] "It borders on irresponsibility. ... But there is a perception that by hyping up this threat you draw people's attention." O'Brien, a former CNN science correspondent, also lamented the lack of television health and science expertise: "Science coverage is important. ... Why in this world where climate change is a big issue, Ebola is a big issue, missing airplanes are a big issue, why is it big entities don't maintain science units anymore? They're gone!"

When Western media outlets did go to West Africa to cover the larger Ebola story firsthand, many drew criticism for their portrayal of the disease and its victims from a foreign perspective. Columbia University journalism professor Howard French[25] sent a letter signed by over 150 academics to the US television network CBS complaining about an Ebola segment on its "60 Minutes" broadcast:

> Africans were reduced to the role of silent victims. They constituted what might be called a scenery of misery. ... Liberians not only died from Ebola, but many of them contributed bravely to the fight against the disease, including doctors, nurses and other caregivers, some of whom gave their lives in this effort. Despite this, the only people heard from on the air were white foreigners who had come to Liberia to contribute to the fight against the disease.

Within West African countries, delays in getting Ebola information to the citizens there also posed a problem. Wade C.L. Williams,[26] an investigative journalist in Liberia, wrote that the panic-stricken government delayed declaring a full state of emergency for four months: "Fear, misinformation and flat-out denial have been far too common ... Among the government's first reactions was to limit journalists' coverage of it. That, in my view, is a major reason the virus has spread as fast as it has ... The effect was to quarantine information about the disease, rather than spread information about how people could protect themselves."

Improving Risk Communication

The news media often do an inadequate job of communicating complex information involving risk, uncertainty, and options for preventive or remedial action. But here again, key stakeholders in the medical, public health, government, political, and private sectors generally do a poor job in communicating risk.

Risk is a three-legged stool involving risk analysis (What is the problem?), risk management (What can be done about the problem?), and risk communication (What should we say to the public?). The first two—analysis and management—get the lion's share of effort from public and private authorities. However, risk communication is often an afterthought rather than a professional discipline requiring training and preparation in its own right. (This is not to be confused with media "spin" by parties more interested in manipulating a message for their own purposes than crafting a clear message to improve public understanding in a crisis.)

For more than three decades, researchers in psychology and communication have sought to understand what drives public concern about health, environmental and technological risks.[27] The conventional wisdom was that providing facts and numbers should persuade the public to agree with experts' assessment of the largest problems. However, studies found that public perception of risk often did not fit this fact-based model.

Simply providing more information, generally through the media, did not necessarily change people's minds or behaviors. Emotional and cognitive factors were at play, with greater concern about risks that were imposed, unfamiliar, uncertain, or catastrophic. (Flying is often incorrectly seen as more dangerous than driving, for example.) Lack of trust also increased concern.

Even though their individual chance of exposure was exceptionally low, people in Texas were more likely to be alarmed about the arrival of a deadly, exotic disease like Ebola and less likely to be worried about everyday dangers of driving, drinking, or getting sick from seasonal influenza.

Journalism's focus on the novel rather than the norm often prods the public to worry about the wrong things. As *Guardian* writer James Ball concluded: "It's worth reflecting what the biggest threat to our collective wellbeing is: rare tropical diseases, or our terrible coverage of them?"[28]

Risk communication and media coverage of infectious disease epidemics can be improved if health authorities learn to craft more useful and timely messages containing accurate, transparent, and relevant public information. News outlets can convey more meaningful risk information by enhancing stories with multimedia images, video, graphics, and interactive tools.

The following ten tips offer strategies for improving global communication and media coverage of public health risks from EVD and other infectious disease epidemics.

1. *Increase media training and risk communication skills for professionals—in public health, medicine, research, government policy, politics, or other fields—who deal with the press and the public in a health crisis.* Increasingly, the public and private sectors are stepping up advance media and crisis management training, using simulation exercises, one-on-one interviews, and video feedback. Content matters, but so does how you look and say it. Transparency builds trust. Accuracy is key but so is acknowledging uncertainty. The media today are democratic: Few people will be professional journalists, but everyone can and should be better communicators.
2. *Know your audience: Who is at greatest risk of exposure to a given harm?* Contracting Ebola requires exposure to the virus: Thus, alarm those at greatest risk of being exposed and calm down those at least risk. Too often experts and media hype generalized or universal messages that get everyone alarmed. Directed messages toward those at greatest risk should provide clear actions to prevent or minimize the danger of new infections, whether in community or health care settings. Conversely, calming down communities or individuals at virtually no risk is important in reducing fear and inappropriate panic. During the Dallas Ebola scare, news photos showed a man wearing a hospital mask while taking out his garbage—a completely unnecessary action.
3. *Provide clear and concise messages about how an infectious disease is or is not transmitted.* The Ebola virus is spread through intimate personal contact with blood or other body fluids in a symptomatic patient, not through the air (as some scaremongers suggested). The incubation period for EVD symptoms to appear is 2 to 21 days after exposure. This silent waiting period increases uncertainty and anxiety. Troubling new studies suggest that survivors can still transmit the Ebola virus sexually after the disease symptoms are gone.
4. *Fight fear with user-friendly facts.* To combat rising Ebola hysteria, the Gannett media chain's television stations and newspapers in the United States mounted an impressive campaign.[29] Using detailed data

from the federal Centers for Disease Control, they partnered to post in-depth Ebola "explainers" on their websites, as well as interactive maps, videos, live chats with experts, and Twitter promotion with the hash tag #FactsNotFear. On the first anniversary of the Texas case, *USA Today* did extensive follow-up stories. Many journalists and commentators sought to put the Ebola risk in perspective, noting that seasonal influenza kills thousands of Americans annually, yet less than half of adults get flu shots.

5. *Remember, "Perception is reality."* Facts alone may not be persuasive enough for some individuals or groups to change their actions or behavior. Recognize that there is no single "public." A given audience reads, watches and listens through multiple lenses of age, gender, ethnicity, education, geography, politics, and religion. But we often act as if there were a generic "public." A variety of emotional and psychological factors may have a greater influence on how danger is perceived and what can be done about it than facts alone. Consider the diversity of the audience.
6. *Put EVD numbers in international perspective.* As of September 20, 2015, the toll from the current West African epidemic numbered 28,331 cases and 11,310 deaths.[30] Of those, only about 24 cases and five deaths were outside of Africa (including 10 cases and two deaths in the United States and the rest in Europe, most of whom were health and aid workers in West Africa who returned home to their countries for treatment).[31] By mid-October 2015, the West African epidemic had waned to only five or fewer cases per week. But Ebola's impact is far from over.[32] Many of the 13,000-plus West African survivors have lingering health problems[33] and live in poverty-stricken countries with struggling health systems and economies further devastated by the latest Ebola onslaught. Careful monitoring for new Ebola cases suggests that even when the disease seems to have disappeared—and countries declared Ebola-free—additional cases may continue to crop up. Out of sight is not necessarily out of harm's way.
7. *Choose risk numbers carefully.* Differentiate relative and absolute risk. Public health studies often use relative risk numbers, finding that a given action or exposure increases the hazard by a given amount—say, a three-fold increase in getting infected. But in order to understand the significance of that relative risk, it is important to know the

baseline, or absolute risk, in the first place. If the risk is 1 in 10,000 to start with, a three-fold increased risk rises to 3 in 10,000—still a small risk. Not all published studies provide the baseline numbers; experts should provide the relevant numbers and members of the news media need to ask.

8. *Avoid inflammatory words.* Using inflammatory words in a public health emergency will of course fan the flames of concern and fear. Ebola is scary enough to start with: Words such as infectious, epidemic, deadly, and quarantine need to be used appropriately. "Catastrophe" and "catastrophic" were often used—from the WHO to CNN—to stress possible consequences, but these words also promoted a doomsday scenario that fed international hysteria. A headline on a WHO six-month update of the epidemic asked, "Ebola in West Africa: Headed for Catastrophe?"[34]
9. *Watch out for seesaw coverage.* A *Washington Post* colleague once quipped that there were two kinds of front-page medical stories: "No hope" and "New hope." Journalists often emphasize the dramatic over the ordinary, but so do experts. In 2014, health and government officials painted an increasingly dire picture of the devastating West African Ebola epidemic. However, many swung toward great optimism when a preliminary 2015 study in the journal *Lancet*[35] reported that human trials in Guinea of a new Ebola vaccine had proven "100 percent" effective. "This new vaccine, if the results hold up, may be the silver bullet against Ebola," waxed Norway's foreign minister Børge Brende.[36] Words such as "silver bullet" or "breakthrough" should generally be avoided. They tend to overpromise solutions that usually take far more time to test and bring to market.
10. *Distinguish personal risk from societal risk.* The news media provide a bullhorn for global awareness of emerging disease threats at the local, national or international level. When the WHO declared Ebola a Public Health Emergency of International Concern in August 2014, it was a belated SOS to the world. The global societal risk was high, requiring immediate support—in manpower and money—to help affected West African nations in caring for patients and communities, while reducing possible spread, particularly into adjacent parts of Africa. But the global personal risk to individual citizens around the world was always

extremely low. Both the societal and personal Ebola risks were very high in many parts of West Africa.

The biggest challenge ahead is keeping public attention focused not only on ending this lingering Ebola virus disease epidemic but also getting better prepared for the next public health emergency, EVD or otherwise. It's not a question of "if," but "when."

"The biggest threat we face now isn't the Ebola virus—it's our short attention span. Whether fueled by apathy, boredom or both, the public's short attention span imperils public health both in developing nations and in the United States," said Dr. Bruce Ribner,[37] director of the Emory Serious Communicable Diseases Unit.

His unit's successful treatment of four Ebola cases from West Africa demonstrated that, although there is no cure, the disease could be managed with sophisticated, supportive care of the kind not available in West Africa. Now he and others at US medical facilities have joined forces with federal health officials to help improve emergency preparedness for future infectious disease threats.

"I'm often asked when the next outbreak will be, and I always say that I can promise you two things: There will be another infectious disease emergency in the next few years, and it won't be a disease we anticipated. The 'next Ebola' probably won't be Ebola at all," said Ribner.

"Each state and locality should have an epidemic response plan. What happens when you fail to plan is that you get caught up in the hysteria, and then politics rules," said Lawrence Gostin,[38] director of the O'Neill Institute for National and Global Health Law at Georgetown University in Washington.

Future emergency preparedness for infectious disease outbreaks should include risk communication and media training as a key pillar, not an afterthought. That includes making better risk communication resources available not only to public health and medical experts but to public information officers, the media, and the public.

At the same time, journalism programs, professional organizations, and mainstream media outlets need to improve training not only of health and science reporters but also of a new generation of general assignment journalists nimble enough to understand and interpret information about emerging infectious diseases. In addition, as the historic Ebola outbreak made clear, the twenty-first century poses new communication challenges and opportunities in a world increasingly connected by travel and technology.

Media coverage of the recent Ebola epidemic illustrates the challenges involved in communicating to the public about a deadly infectious disease. The media shares much of the blame for the hyperbole that surrounded Ebola, especially its limited arrival in America. But there were countless mistakes among many stakeholders in the communication supply chain, especially those who jumped in and politicized the Ebola epidemic, fanning the flames of public concern. What's needed going forward is a proactive effort by the public health community to improve communication to the media as well as the public. Responsible media also share the responsibility to be more prepared and knowledgeable for the next international disease epidemic.

We should all be expecting it.

Notes

1. "Ebola Virus in Guinea," World Health Organization Africa, Regional Office, accessed September 28, 2015, http://www.afro.who.int/pt/grupos-organicos-e-programas/ddc/alerta-e-resposta-epidemias-e-pandemias/4063-ebola-hemorrhagic-fever-in-guinea.html.

2. "Outbreaks Chronology, Ebola Virus Disease," Centers for Disease Control and Prevention, accessed September 28, 2015, http://www.cdc.gov/vhf/ebola/outbreaks/history/chronology.html.

3. "Ebola virus disease, West Africa—update 4 August 2014," World Health Organization Africa, Regional Office, http://www.afro.who.int/en/clusters-a-programmes/dpc/epidemic-a-pandemic-alert-and-response/outbreak-news/4239-ebola-virus-disease-west-africa-4-august-2014.html.

4. Scott Gordon, "Ebola Patient Dr. Kent Brantly Discharged, Cured of Deadly Disease," *NBCDFW.com*, August 21, 2014, accessed September 27, 2015, http://www.nbcdfw.com/news/health/Ebola-Patient-Dr-Kent-Brantly-to-Leave-Hospital-Thursday-272102161.html.

5. "WHO Virtual Press Conference following the Meeting of the International Health Regulations Emergency Committee regarding the 2014 Ebola Outbreak in West Africa," World Health Organization, August 8, 2014, http://www.who.int/mediacentre/multimedia/2014/who-ebola-outbreak-08aug2014.pdf?ua=1.

6. "Barriers to rapid containment of the Ebola outbreak: Ebola situation assessment," World Health Organization, August 11, 2014, http://www.who.int/mediacentre/news/ebola/overview-august-2014/en/.

7. Manny Fernandez and Julie Bosman, "Ebola Victim's Family Blames Hospital and State," *New York Times,* October 11, 2014, http://www.nytimes.com/2014/10/12/us/ebola-victims-family-blames-hospital-and-state.html.

8. Brenda Goodman, "Ebola Patient in Dallas, Thomas Eric Duncan, Dies," *WebMD Health News*, October 7, 2014, http://www.webmd.com/news/20141008/dallas-ebola-patient-duncan.

9. "Sierra Leone Records 121 Ebola Deaths, 81 New Cases in Single Day," *NBCNews.com,* October 6, 2014, http://www.nbcnews.com/storyline/ebola-virus-outbreak/sierra-leone-records-121-ebola-deaths-81-new-cases-single-n219151.

10. Emily Thomas, "This Illustration of Ebola Coverage Shows How Problematic Media Reports Can Be," *Huffington Post,* October 8, 2014, http://www.huffingtonpost.com/2014/10/08/ebola-illustration-andre-carrilho_n_5955192.html.

11. Brady Dennis and Peyton M. Craighill, "Ebola Poll: Two-Thirds of Americans Worried about Possible Widespread Epidemic in U.S.," *Washington Post,* October 14, 2014, https://www.washingtonpost.com/national/health-science/ebola-poll-two-thirds-of-americans-worried-about-possible-widespread-epidemic-in-us/2014/10/13/d0afd0ee-52ff-11e4-809b-8cc0a295c773_story.html.

12. Chico Harlan, "An Epidemic of Fear and Anxiety Hits Americans Amid Ebola Outbreak," *Washington Post,* October 15, 2014, http://www.washingtonpost.com/business/economy/an-epidemic-of-fear-and-anxiety-hits-americans-amid-ebola-outbreak/2014/10/15/0760fb96-54a8-11e4-ba4b-f6333e2c0453_story.html.

13. Kathleen O'Brien, "Ebola Poll: N.J. Residents Fear An Outbreak in the U.S., but Aren't Well Informed about the Disease," *NJ.com,* October 9, 2015, http://www.nj.com/healthfit/index.ssf/2014/10/ebola_poll_nj_fears_an_outbreak_here.html.

14. "2014 West African Ebola Outbreak: Feature Map," World Health Organization, accessed September 27, 2015, http://www.who.int/features/ebola/storymap/en/. "Ebola Virus Disease, Fact Sheet," World Health Organization, August 2015, accessed September 27, 2015, http://www.who.int/entity/mediacentre/factsheets/fs103/en/.

15. Michele Dean, "Back in the Hot Zone: What to Read about Ebola," *The Guardian,* October 28, 2014, http://www.theguardian.com/books/2014/oct/28/what-to-read-about-ebola-books.

16. Centers for Disease Control and Prevention, "Outbreaks Chronology, Ebola Virus Disease."

17. "Ebola Crisis: "WHO Signals Help for Africa to Stop Spread," *BBC.com*, October 16, 2014, http://www.bbc.com/news/world-africa-29648598.

18. Ken White, "Media Coverage of Ebola Requires a Delicate Balance," *Poynter.org,* October 5, 2014, http://www.poynter.org/how-tos/leadership-management/272907/media-coverage-of-ebola-requires-a-delicate-balance/.

19. "Times Coverage of Ebola: Pulitzer-Winning Articles and More," *New York Times,* April 20, 2015, http://www.nytimes.com/interactive/2015/04/20/world/africa/ebola-coverage-pulitzer.html.

20. Paul Farhi, "Media Goes Overtime on Ebola Coverage, but Not Necessarily Overboard," *Washington Post,* October 6, 2014, https://www.washingtonpost.com/lifestyle/style/media-goes-overtime-on-ebola-coverage-but-not-necessarily-overboard/2014/10/06/d65e92fc-4d8a-11e4-8c24-487e92bc997b_story.html.

21. Cristine Russell, "Here's How to Produce Strong Ebola Stories," *Columbia Journalism Review,* October 6, 2014, http://www.cjr.org/the_observatory/ebola_science_reporters_are_im.php.

22. "Top doctor 'Not Surprised' if US Has Another Ebola Case, Downplays Use of Virus in Bioterror Attack," *FoxNews.com,* October 5, 2014, http://www.foxnews.com/politics/2014/10/05/fauci-not-surprised-if-us-has-another-ebola-case-virus-smuggled-across-mexico/.

23. Joe Coscarelli, "Ebola Coverage Goes Extra Dumb on CNN, Fox News," *New York Magazine,* October 6, 2014, http://nymag.com/daily/intelligencer/2014/10/ebola-coverage-extra-dumb-cnn-fox-news.html#. "CNN Calls Ebola 'ISIS of biological agents' after accusing FOX of being unscientific," Youtube.com, October 6, 2014, accessed September 28, 2015, https://www.youtube.com/watch?v=aOMgenA56Ao.

24. Evan McMurry, "Science Reporter Slams Fox's Ebola Coverage: 'Level of Ignorance We Shouldn't Allow in Media,'" *Mediaite.com,* October 5, 2014, http://www.mediaite.com/tv/science-reporter-slams-foxs-ebola-coverage-level-of-ignorance-we-shouldnt-allow-in-media/.

25. Howard French, "The worst of journalism: 200 writers and academics slam CBS coverage of Africa," *The Guardian,* March 26, 2015, http://www.theguardian.com/world/2015/mar/26/cbs-africa-howard-french; Howard French, "How Does Africa Get Reported? A Letter of Concern to 60 Minutes," A Glimpse of the World (blog), March 26, 2015, accessed September 27, 2015, http://www.howardwfrench.com/2015/03/how-does-africa-get-reported-a-letter-of-concern-to-60-minutes/.

26. Wade C. L. Williams, "In the Grip of Ebola," *The New York Times,* August 7, 2014, http://www.nytimes.com/2014/08/08/opinion/in-the-grip-of-ebola.html.

27. There are numerous background books on risk communication. Here are a few: Baruch Fischhoff and John Kadvany, *Risk: A Very Short Introduction* (New York: Oxford University Press, 2011); Robert L. Heath & H. Dan O'Hair, Eds. *Handbook of Risk Perception* (New York: Routledge, 2010); David Ropeik, *How Risky Is It, Really? Why Our Fears Don't Always Match the Facts* (McGraw Hill Education, 2010); National Research Council, *Improving Risk Communication* (Washington, DC: National Academy Press, 1989).

28. James Ball, "Concerned about Ebola? You're Worrying about the Wrong Disease," *The Guardian,* August 5, 2014, http://www.theguardian.com/commentisfree/2014/aug/05/ebola-worrying-disease.

29. David Uberti, "Media Changes Course on Ebola," *Columbia Journalism Review,* October 17, 2014, http://www.cjr.org/behind_the_news/media_changes_course_on_ebola.php.

30. World Health Organization, "Ebola Situation Report—23 September 2015," accessed September 28, 2015, http://apps.who.int/ebola/current-situation/ebola-situation-report-23-september-2015.

31. "How Many Ebola Patients Have Been Treated outside of Africa?" *The New York Times,* January 26, 2015, http://www.nytimes.com/interactive/2014/07/31/world/africa/ebola-virus-outbreak-qa.html.

32. World Health Organization, "Ebola Situation Report—21 October 2015," accessed October 23, 2015, http://apps.who.int/ebola/current-situation/ebola-situation-report-21-october-2015.

33. Denise Grady, "Ebola Survivors Face Lingering Pain, Fatigue, and Depression," *The New York Times,* August 7, 2015, http://www.nytimes.com/2015/08/08/health/ebola-survivors-face-lingering-pain-fatigue-and-depression.html.

34. "Ebola in West Africa: Heading for Catastrophe?," WHO website, accessed September 28, 2015, http://www.who.int/csr/disease/ebola/ebola-6-months/west-africa/en/.

35. "An Ebola Vaccine: First Results and Promising Opportunities," *The Lancet* 382 (2015), 830, doi: 10.1016/S0140-6736(15)61177-1.

36. Sarah Bosely, "Ebola Vaccine Trial Proves 100% Effective in Guinea," *The Guardian,* July 31, 2015, http://www.theguardian.com/world/2015/jul/31/ebola-vaccine-trial-proves-100-successful-in-guinea.

37. Bruce Ribner, "The Biggest Infectious Disease Threat We Face Isn't Ebola—It's Our Short Attention Span," The Conversation, August 12, 2015, accessed September 27, 2015, https://theconversation.com/the-biggest-infectious-disease-threat-we-face-isnt-ebola-its-our-short-attention-span-45544.

38. Liz Szabo, "Some Health Experts Say the USA Hasn't Learned Key Lessons from Ebola Experience," *USA Today,* September 22, 2015, http://www.usatoday.com/story/news/2015/09/22/some-health-experts-say-usa-hasnt-learned-key-lessons-ebola-experience/72538614/.

12 When Reassurance Doesn't Reassure: Reporters, Sources, and Ebola in Dallas

Marjorie Kruvand

As Ebola in West Africa dominated global news coverage during the spring and summer of 2014, federal officials repeatedly offered assurances that the American health system was well equipped to seamlessly handle the virus if it arrived on US soil.[1] President Barack Obama weighed in, saying several times that he had confidence in the US Centers for Disease Control and Prevention (CDC).[2] But when a patient died of Ebola virus disease (EVD) at Texas Health Presbyterian Hospital (Presbyterian) in Dallas, Texas, after a botched diagnosis, and two nurses there also became infected, public confidence in CDC plummeted.[3]

CDC Director Thomas R. Frieden acknowledged at a news conference on October 14, 2014, that the agency should have responded sooner to the first case in Dallas and done more to prevent additional infections.[4] Those comments marked an about-face in the tone of CDC's communication: The agency that had appeared so confident about its preparedness to handle Ebola in the United States was now contrite about its missteps. CDC officials were lampooned in editorial cartoons for a lack of credibility and criticized in news stories for offering conflicting advice—and sometimes no timely advice at all—about how to prevent the spread of the virus.[5]

Previous chapters have discussed the public health messages disseminated during the Ebola outbreak and how they were delivered to the public through the news and social media. But what about the senders of those messages? Who did journalists rely on as sources of information about Ebola in the United States? How did their communication, or lack of timely communication, aid or harm the situation? Did they help, clarify, or confuse? Reassure or alarm? And how could they have communicated more effectively?

These questions matter because the public gets much of its information about health and science from the news media.[6] The news media serve as brokers between health, science, and the public, shaping public consciousness about events and helping to set the agenda for public policy.[7] The news media also forcefully shape how policy issues related to health and scientific controversies are defined, symbolized, and resolved.[8]

Americans were drawn to media coverage of Ebola at historically high rates.[9] Nearly half of US adults (49 percent) reported that they followed news about the outbreak very closely in mid-October 2014, up from 26 percent in early August 2014.[10] The only news topics that drew more attention in the United States during the previous two years were the Boston Marathon bombing (63 percent), the 2012 Congressional election (60 percent), the school shootings in Newtown, Connecticut (57 percent), and Hurricane Sandy (53 percent).[11]

Journalists and Sources

Newsgathering is a collective activity in which journalists depend on others—and especially on official sources—for much of the content of their stories.[12] In turn, journalists' choice of sources significantly influences how their stories are shaped and told.[13] Health and science reporters tend to turn to a relatively small roster of sources: scientists, physicians, government and industry officials, and bioethicists.[14] Reporters work most efficiently when they know in advance what the sources they plan to interview will say.[15] Journalists thus develop a small cadre of "go–to" sources on whom they can rely to provide certain information or the opinion needed to complete a story.[16] Reporters "find it easier and more predictable to consult a narrow range of experts than to call on new ones each time."[17] Sources with highly visible names, titles, affiliations, and even a touch of celebrity are prized.[18]

Journalists need sources for information, explanation, context, implications, and opinion. But what journalists really *want* from sources is accessibility; exclusivity; rapid response; quotes that are pithy, colorful, and memorable; and comments that promote controversy and sensationalism.[19] In other words, journalists would like public health officials, scientists, and physicians to communicate in ways antithetical to their professional training. That's because of the differences among the fields of science, medicine, and journalism and the missions of physicians, scientists, public health officials, and journalists.

While science and medicine are "slow, precise, careful, conservative and complicated," journalism is "hungry for headlines and drama, fast, short, dramatic, (and) very imprecise at times."[20] Scientists, physicians, and public health officials care greatly about context, precision, qualification, and nuance.[21] In contrast, journalists care about timeliness, accuracy, balance, and, above all, getting a story—the bigger and juicier the better.[22] As a result, journalists may ferret out inconsistencies in what a source says, challenge discrepancies between sources, question pat answers, and criticize slow response or lack of response.

Three official sources—CDC Director Thomas R. Frieden; Dr. Daniel Varga, chief clinical officer of Texas Health Resources, Presbyterian's parent company; and Dallas County Judge Clay Jenkins—prominently figured in news coverage of Ebola in Dallas. Frieden is a physician and former New York City health commissioner who has been CDC director since 2009.[23] Varga joined Texas Health Resources in 2013 as its first chief clinical officer.[24] Jenkins is Dallas County's chief executive and its director of homeland security and emergency management.[25]

Inform and Reassure

Americans have near-record low levels of trust in the federal government.[26] Only 24 percent of Americans surveyed say they can trust the federal government to do what is right nearly all or most of the time, while 75 percent say they trust the government only some of the time or never.[27] After the often-frenetic news coverage about the Ebola outbreak in West Africa, which both reflected and magnified public fear and uncertainty, CDC's initial approach to communication about Ebola in the United States was to inform and reassure. Frieden told journalists in August 2014 that US hospitals were ready if Ebola surfaced in America:

> CDC officials have said repeatedly that any hospital in the United States can safely provide care for a patient with Ebola by following their exacting infection-control procedures and isolating the patient in a private room with an unshared bathroom. "What's needed to fight Ebola is not fancy equipment," Frieden said. "What's needed is standard infection control, rigorously applied."[28]

But these reassuring words ultimately rang hollow at Presbyterian. For weeks, the hospital was the epicenter of the Ebola story in the United States after Thomas Eric Duncan, a Liberian man who became ill while visiting relatives in Dallas, went to the emergency room with a high fever on September 26, 2014, but was sent home without being diagnosed with EVD.[29] Duncan returned by ambulance two days later after his symptoms worsened. He was diagnosed with EVD on September 30, two days after he was admitted.[30]

Even after Duncan's case was confirmed, US health officials continued to play down fears of Ebola.[31] Frieden told reporters that methods to track down people who may have been exposed to Ebola through contact with Duncan were "tried and true," adding, "I have no doubt that we'll stop this in its tracks in the U.S."[32] At the same time, however, news stories noted that health officials had delayed for more than a week the cleanup of the Dallas apartment where Duncan had stayed with relatives before entering the hospital, leaving potentially infectious bedding and other items in place.[33]

Frieden also said there was no reason to move Duncan to another hospital, reiterating that any US hospital capable of isolating patients for other infectious diseases could safely handle Ebola cases.[34] And Presbyterian's epidemiologist, Dr. Edward Goodman, told reporters: "We have had a plan in place for some time now for a patient presenting with possible Ebola. ... We were well prepared to care for this patient."[35]

Duncan died at Presbyterian on October 8, the first Ebola fatality in the United States. His death would have been major news in itself, but media attention magnified after two nurses who cared for Duncan also contracted EVD. News stories described those new infections as "the straw that broke the camel's back," diminishing public confidence in how Ebola was being handled in Dallas.[36]

Journalists also complained that Presbyterian initially provided scant additional information to the media:

> Presbyterian has routinely refused requests from ... news organizations to provide more information about the Duncan case and the subsequent infections. Even general questions about the record-keeping system have been ignored—or are indefinitely "under consideration" for a response—and the strategy seems to primarily include offering as little information as possible.[37]

Lack of communication opened Presbyterian to even more media scrutiny and criticism. News stories described Presbyterian as "a hospital under siege" after "a cascade of mishaps"[38] and as experiencing "a nightmare without end."[39]

When the two nurses with Ebola were moved to hospitals in other states for treatment, news stories highlighted the inherent mixed messages. On one hand, the moves meant that the nurses no longer presented a risk of infection to co-workers, other patients, or the community. On the other hand, it signaled that despite Presbyterian's repeated claims that it had been prepared for Ebola and CDC's assurances that any hospital could safely handle Ebola cases, Presbyterian was deemed incapable of offering its own nurses the best possible treatment.[40] Both nurses recovered.

Two national public opinion polls released on October 21, 2014, showed a simultaneous increase in public concern over Ebola and a decline in trust in government officials managing Ebola in the United States.[41] A survey by the Pew Research Center found that 41 percent of Americans said they were worried that they or someone in their families would be exposed to the virus, up from 32 percent two weeks earlier. Meanwhile, a Gallup poll showed a decline in Americans' confidence in the "federal government's ability to handle Ebola" from 60 percent to 52 percent in a single week.[42] Those numbers raised the communication stakes even higher.

Judgment Questioned

Official sources, including Frieden, Varga, and Jenkins, attempted to assure the community—and beyond—that Ebola was under control in Dallas, but their confidence did not square with what people were reading, seeing, and hearing in the news. For example, 75 Presbyterian employees involved in Duncan's care were ordered to stay home and monitor themselves for Ebola symptoms,[43] several schools in Texas and Ohio were closed temporarily,[44] and Frontier Airlines replaced carpeting and seat covers on two planes on which a nurse infected with Ebola virus had flown.[45]

Some communication efforts in Dallas appeared awkward or even counterproductive. For example, in an ABC News story headlined "Ebola Scare Turns Dallas Hospital into a 'Ghost Town,'" Varga was quoted as saying:

I would tell this community that Presby [the hospital's nickname] is an absolutely safe hospital to come to. We've been in communication with our doctors that have private offices in our professional buildings around the campus who are getting 40, 50, 60 percent cancellations just for fear of being somewhere in the geography of the hospital where Ebola is treated.[46]

But reporters—and through their stories, the public—believed Presbyterian was the opposite of "absolutely safe":

Long regarded as one of the finest hospitals in Texas, Presbyterian has faced continuing criticism—first for its initial misdiagnosis of Mr. Duncan, which delayed his care and placed others at risk; then for issuing contradictory statements about why its doctors did not suspect Ebola; and now for failures in safety protocol that led to the infections of two of its own. If the hospital has served as a canary in a coal mine for the country's Ebola response, the results have not inspired confidence.[47]

Stories included criticism from a national nurses union and even some Presbyterian employees that Duncan's case had been handled sloppily, putting health care workers and other patients at risk of infection.[48] NPR reported that hospital managers "first seemed unsure what sort of protection should be worn. Eventually, it settled on caps, particulate masks, face shields and goggles. That left parts of the head and neck exposed. It wasn't until ... Duncan was finally confirmed by the CDC as positive for Ebola that the hospital issued fully hooded hazmat suits."[49]

Presbyterian leaders said that in caring for Duncan, the hospital had followed CDC's initial guidance on what health care workers treating Ebola patients should wear:

CDC says that health care workers ... need only wear gloves, a fluid-resistant gown, eye protection and a face mask to prevent becoming infected with the virus. That is a far cry from the head-to-toe "moon suits" doctors, nurses and aides have been seeing on television reports about the outbreak.[50]

After Duncan's death and the infection of two nurses, Presbyterian and CDC strengthened their guidelines on protective clothing. But media criticism of Presbyterian also focused on the hospital's leadership:

This failure of judgment put the lives of its medical staff and especially its nurses at risk. ... Here was a recently traveled patient from West Africa exhibiting effusive and classic symptoms of Ebola. It was senseless not to provide the medical staff with the best protection the hospital had on hand. Varga admits Presbyterian wasn't ready. They hadn't trained for Ebola and were not wise enough about the threat the virus posed.[51]

When CDC belatedly flooded Presbyterian with teams of infection-control experts and crisis managers after Duncan's death, Frieden acknowledged that the agency should have responded more quickly and aggressively.[52] "I wish we had put a team like this on the ground the day the patient, the first patient, was diagnosed," he said. "That might have prevented this infection. But we will do that from today onward with any case, anywhere in the U.S."[53]

Acknowledging its missteps marked the beginning of CDC's efforts to rebuild public trust. Presbyterian was also ready to apologize and attempt to move on. But after a series of contradictory news releases, inaccurate statements, unanswered questions, and growing criticism over how Duncan was treated,[54] damage to the hospital's reputation was so extensive that Texas Health Resources hired Burson-Marsteller, a public relations agency, to help conduct "an aggressive public relations campaign aimed at rehabilitating its battered image."[55] A few days later, Texas Health Resources bought full-page newspaper ads in Dallas and Fort Worth to apologize for not living up to "the high standards that are the heart of our hospital's history, mission and commitment" by botching Duncan's initial diagnosis.[56]

Varga was out front in the "public relations offensive to restore trust."[57] In prepared Congressional testimony, he said: "Despite our best intentions and a highly skilled medical team, we made mistakes. We did not correctly diagnose his symptoms as those of Ebola. We are deeply sorry."[58] Presbyterian also flooded social media with the hashtag "#PresbyProud" to try to staunch the number of patients continuing to stay away.[59] And Presbyterian scored a media relations coup when former President George W. Bush, a former patient, visited employees and patients at the hospital.[60] But news stories panned the stage-managed quality of some of Presbyterian's public relations activities, which undermined their credibility:

> The hospital published slick video clips of smiling nurses praising their managers and hosted a brief "rally" of medics wielding pro-hospital placards outside the emergency room for television news cameras. The placards, bearing such slogans as 'We (heart) Presby' and 'We stand with Presby,' appeared to have been written in the same handwriting.[61]

Communication Lessons Learned

How could official sources—and the organizations they represent—have communicated more effectively with the public through the news media about Ebola in the United States? Principles of risk and crisis communication provide several suggestions.

First, communicate early and often, even when not all the facts are known. For example, when Presbyterian provided scant information to journalists after two of its nurses were diagnosed with Ebola, it violated a tenet of crisis communication: If you don't fill the information vacuum, someone else will.[62] In Presbyterian's case, the "someone else" included members of Congress, pundits on cable television networks, a national nurses union, Duncan's relatives and neighbors, and personal injury lawyers, all of whom used the news media as a platform to air their views—including criticism of Presbyterian's handling of Ebola.

Second, statements meant to reassure the public can backfire, especially when they are at odds with what is really happening. Crisis communication expert Peter M. Sandman suggests that officials be "as reassuring as you can be so long as you are virtually certain that reality won't turn out worse than your reassurances."[63] But as the *Los Angeles Times* noted in an editorial on the CDC's handling of Ebola: "In an attempt to avoid a public panic, they instead created a worse one by making assurances that were quickly shown to be wrong. … It looked as though government experts weren't in control, and that sparked fear."[64]

Sandman notes that empty reassurance isn't reassuring,[65] a point also made in several editorials on Ebola in the United States:

> Even as U.S. health authorities continue to tell Americans not to worry about the Ebola virus, their assurances are being undercut by the increasingly obvious deficiencies in domestic planning. … Frieden … has repeatedly been forced to back away from his calming assertions that U.S. hospitals were ready for the disease.[66]

USA Today editorialized that while CDC "is known for providing calm expertise in a health crisis," Frieden at times "let overconfidence get ahead of facts": "CDC allowed its desire to tamp down fear to 'get ahead of the science,' said infectious disease specialist Michael Osterholm."[67]

Sandman also cautions officials to never proclaim that anything is "safe."[68] Varga's comment that Presbyterian was "absolutely safe" not only failed to reassure, but also prompted journalists to catalog in news stories the many ways they believed the hospital was unsafe.

Third, sources—and the organizations they represent—should actively safeguard their trustworthiness. Credibility is a source's most important asset, and if it is challenged or eroded, their information or opinion is much less likely to be sought by reporters, included in media coverage, and attended to by the public. Sandman points out that one way in which trust can be diminished is over-reassurance: "People sense that you're withholding alarming information and become all the more fearful. Or they learn later that you withheld alarming information and never trust you again."[69]

Fourth, being defensive, dodging responsibility, or attempting to shift the blame to others can hinder crisis recovery.[70] In November 2014, Presbyterian officials still maintained that the hospital had been prepared for Ebola despite every indication to the contrary over the previous five weeks. Varga told a public forum in Dallas: "We were completely and adequately prepared to treat a patient with Ebola but less than completely prepared for a patient to come in from the streets and for us to give diagnosis of Ebola."[71] Either Presbyterian was prepared or it wasn't; anything else is splitting hairs.

Fifth, empathy should be an essential part of communication. Public opinion is shaped by emotion as well as reason, and demonstrating public health expertise isn't enough when emotions run high. As risk communication expert Dr. Vincent T. Covello asserts: "When people are stressed and upset, they want to know that you care before they care what you know."[72]

Expressions of empathy can humanize officials and make their words more believable. Officials could have demonstrated empathy during the Ebola crisis in the United States by acknowledging publicly that they understood why people were upset and frightened—even if they personally believed there was no rational reason for people to feel that way. Although the number of Ebola cases in the United States was small, the number of Americans worried about, and inconvenienced by, Ebola was considerably larger. Yet there was no public recognition of the anxiety experienced by health care workers who may have been put in harm's way by lax safety protocols, the disrupted lives and lost pay of people ordered to stay home and monitor themselves for Ebola symptoms, the inconvenience to parents whose children's schools were closed, and the concern of air travelers who were later told they had flown with an infected passenger.

Jenkins, the Dallas county judge, expressed empathy more effectively than the other official sources in Dallas. He drove Duncan's relatives to a quarantine location and then told a news conference later that day that he was still wearing the same clothes because he was unconcerned about contracting Ebola.[73] As one reporter described Jenkins, "No local, state or federal official involved in the Ebola emergency in Dallas has put himself farther on the front lines and done more to humanize and personalize the government response."[74] Yet the most empathetic moment occurred in Washington, DC—1,300 miles from Dallas—when President Obama hugged Nina Pham in the Oval Office on October 24, 2014.[75] Pham, a nurse at Presbyterian, had been released from an Atlanta hospital earlier that day after recovering from Ebola.

Finally, reputation-repair efforts after a crisis must be perceived as authentic. News stories noted that some of Presbyterian's activities to restore its image and regain patients' trust appeared to be less of a genuine grassroots effort and more of a carefully scripted campaign managed by a major public relations agency, including YouTube videos with high production values, prepared remarks at a news conference at which no questions from reporters were allowed, a brief employee "rally" for the benefit of television cameras, and lack of media access to hospital leaders.[76] Reporters also noted that "a good number" of the tweets with the hashtag #PresbyProud "came from official hospital accounts or from those of top managers."[77]

Moreover, although offering an apology is an important step to regain trust, it isn't enough—especially in a severe or prolonged crisis like Ebola in the Unites States. Crisis communicators assert that communication should follow performance: An organization should fix its problems first, then communicate the changes and improvements to the news media and public, and finally, demonstrate over time that the changes actually work.[78]

In hindsight, applying these principles of risk and crisis communication could have improved public communication through the news media about Ebola in the United States. They may also provide useful guidance during future infectious disease outbreaks.

Notes

1. Manny Fernandez, Michael D. Shear, and Abby Goodnough, "Dallas Hospital Alters Account, Raising Questions on Ebola Case," *The New York Times*, October 3, 2014, http://www.nytimes.com/2014/10/04/us/containing-ebola-cdc-troops-west-africa.html.

2. Ibid.

3. Sarah Dutton, Jennifer De Pinto, Anthony Salvanto, and Fred Backus, "Public Confidence in CDC Nosedives, Poll Finds," CBS News, October 17, 2014, http://www.cbsnews.com/news/cbs-news-poll-confidence-cdc-nosedives-since-ebola.

4. Mark Berman, "CDC Director: We Could Have Done More to Prevent Second Ebola Infection in Texas," *Washington Post*, October 14, 2014, http://www.washingtonpost.com/pb/newssearch/?query=cdc+director%3A+we+could+have+done+more; Manny Fernandez and Jack Healy, "C.D.C. Says it Should Have Responded Faster to the Dallas Ebola Case," *The New York Times*, October 14, 2015, http://www.nytimes.com/2014/10/15/us/cdc-says-it-should-have-responded-more-quickly-to-dallas-ebola-case.html.

5. Laura Keeney, "CDC Dropping Ball on Keeping Public Informed," *Denver Post*, October 18, 2014, 1A.

6. Pew Research Center, "Ebola Ranks among Highest in News Interest Since 2010," October 21, 2014, http://www.pewresearch.org/fact-tank/2014/10/21/ebola-ranks-among-highest-in-news-interest-since-2010/.

7. Dorothy Nelkin, "Beyond Risk: Reporting about Genetics in the Post-Asilomar Press," *Perspectives in Biology and Medicine* 44, no. 2 (2001).

8. Matthew C. Nisbet and Dietram A. Scheufele, "What's Next for Science Communication? Promising Directions and Lingering Distractions," *American Journal of Botany* 96, no. 10 (2009); Matthew C. Nisbet, Dominique Brossard, and Adrianne Kroepsch, "Framing Science: The Stem Cell Controversy in an Age of Press/Politics," *The International Journal of Press/Politics* 8, no. 2 (2003).

9. Pew Research Center, "Ebola Ranks Among Highest in News Interest Since 2010."

10. Ibid.

11. Ibid.

12. Peter Conrad, "Uses of Expertise: Sources, Quotes, and Voice in the Reporting of Genetics in the News," *Public Understanding of Science* 8, no. 4 (1999); Leon V. Sigal, *Reporters and Officials: The Organization and Politics of Newsmaking* (Lexington, MA: Heath, 1973).

13. Scott R. Maier and Twange Kasoma, "Information as Good as its Source—An Examination of Source Diversity and Accuracy at Nine Daily U.S. Newspapers." Paper presented at the annual conference of the International Communication Association, New York, May 2005.

14. Conrad, "Uses of Expertise"; Sharon Dunwoody, "Scientists, Journalists, and the News," *Chemical & Engineering News* 65, no. 46 (1987); Sharon Dunwoody and Michael Ryan, "The Credible Scientific Source," *Journalism Quarterly* 64 (1987);

Rae Goodell, *The Visible Scientists* (Boston: Little, Brown, 1977); Marjorie Kruvand, "Bioethicists as Expert Sources in Science and Medical Reporting," *Newspaper Research Journal* 30, no. 3 (2009); Dorothy Nelkin, *Selling Science: How the Press Covers Science and Technology*. (New York: Freeman, 1995); Nisbet, Brossard and Kroepsch, "Framing Science: The Stem Cell Controversy in an Age of Press/Politics"; Matthew C. Nisbet and Bruce V. Lewenstein, "Biotechnology and the American Media: The Policy Process and the Elite Press, 1970 to 1999," *Science Communication* 23 (2002).

15. Pamela J. Shoemaker and Stephen D. Reese, *Mediating the Message: Theories of Influences on Mass Media Content* (White Plains, NY: Longman, 1996).

16. Conrad, "Uses of Expertise"; Shoemaker and Reese, *Mediating the Message*; Stephen D. Reese, August Grant, and Lucig H. Danielian, "The Structure of News Sources on Television: A Network Analysis of 'CBS News,' 'Nightline,' 'MacNeil/Lehrer' and 'This Week with David Brinkley,' *Journal of Communication* 44, no. 2 (1994).

17. Shoemaker and Reese, *Mediating the Message*, 131.

18. Conrad, "Uses of Expertise"; Julia B. Corbett and Motomi Mori, "Medicine, Media and Celebrities: News Coverage of Breast Cancer, 1960–1995," *Journalism and Mass Communication Quarterly* 76, no. 2 (1999); Goodell, *The Visible Scientists*; Marjorie Kruvand, "'Dr. Soundbite': The Making of an Expert Source in Science and Medical Stories," *Science Communication* 34, no. 5 (2012); Randall S. Sumpter and Johny T. Garner, "Telling the Columbia Story: Source Selection in News Accounts of a Shuttle Accident," *Science Communication* 28, no. 4 (2007).

19. Erik Albaek, Peter M. Christiansen, and Lise Togeby, "Experts in the Mass Media: Researchers as Sources in Danish Daily Newspapers, 1961–2001," *Journalism and Mass Communication Quarterly* 80, no. 4 (2003); Tammy Boyce, "Journalism and Expertise," *Journalism Studies* 7, no. 6 (2006); Kruvand, "Dr. Soundbite."

20. Kathy Sawyer, cited in Jim Hartz and Rick Chappell, "Worlds Apart: How the Distance between Science and Journalism Threatens America's Future," First Amendment Center, Vanderbilt University, 1997, 14, http://www.firstamendmentcenter.org/madison/wp-content/uploads/2011/03/worldsapart.pdf.

21. Jane Gregory and Steve Miller, "Working with the Media," in *Handbook of Science Communication,* ed. Anthony Wilson (Bristol, UK: Institute of Physics Publishing, 1998).

22. Susan Dentzer, "Communicating Medical News—Pitfalls of Health care Journalism," *New England Journal of Medicine* 360, no. 1 (2009).

23. US Centers for Disease Control and Prevention, "The CDC Director," May 17, 2013, http://www.cdc.gov/about/leadership/director.htm.

24. Texas Health Resources, "Bio of Daniel Varga, M.D.," last modified 2015, accessed July 12, 2015, https://www.texashealth.org/pages/Leadership/Daniel-Varga-M-D.aspx.

25. Dallas County, "Bio of Dallas County Judge Clay Jenkins," last modified 2010, accessed July 13, 2015, http://www.dallascounty.org/department/comcrt/jenkins/bio.php.

26. Pew Research Center, "Beyond Red vs. Blue: The Political Typology. Section 2: Views of the Nation, the Constitution and Government," June 26, 2014, accessed July 14, 2015, http://www.people-press.org/2014/06/26/section-2-views-of-the-nation-the-constitution-and-government/#trust.

27. Ibid.

28. Catherine St. Louis, "Hospitals in the U.S. Get Ready for Ebola," *The New York Times*, August 16, 2014, A11.

29. Manny Fernandez and Kevin Sack, "Ebola Patient Sent Home Despite Fever, Records Show," *The New York Times*, October 14, 2014, http://www.nytimes.com/2014/10/11/us/thomas-duncan-had-a-fever-of-103-er-records-show.html.

30. Fernandez and Healy, "C.D.C. Says it Should Have Responded Faster."

31. Sarah Portlock and Alan Zibel, "U.S. Health Officials Continue to Play Down Ebola Fears," *Wall Street Journal*, October 5, 2014, http://www.wsj.com/articles/u-s-health-officials-continue-to-play-down-ebola-fears-1412529955.

32. Denise Grady, "First U.S. Case is Confirmed: Ebola in Texas," *The New York Times*, October 1, 2014, A1.

33. Fernandez, Shear, and Goodnough, "Dallas Hospital Alters Account."

34. Grady, "First U.S. Case is Confirmed."

35. Ibid.

36. Wade Goodwyn, "Dallas Hospital Deals with Aftermath of Ebola Missteps," NPR, October 18, 2014, http://www.npr.org/2014/10/18/357153319/dallas-hospital-deals-with-aftermath-of-ebola-missteps.

37. Nicolas M. Mora and Jim Dalrymple II, "Can Texas Hospital Recover from Ebola Scare?" BuzzFeed, October 22, 2014, http://www.buzzfeed.com/nicolasmedinamora/what-do-you-say-on-when-an-ebola-patient-dies-in-your-hospit#.esDGVWan0.

38. Randy L. Loftis, Sarah Mervosh, and Marc Ramirez, "Ebola Crisis is Testing Presbyterian Hospital Dallas," *Dallas Morning News*, October 18, 2014, http://www.dallasnews.com/business/health-care/20141018-ebola-crisis-is-testing-presbyterian-hospital-dallas.ece.

39. Kevin Sack, "Downfall for Hospital where Ebola Spread," *The New York Times,* October 15, 2014, accessed January 7, 2015, http://www.nytimes.com/2014/10/16/us/infamy-for-dallas-hospital-where-virus-spread.html.

40. Goodwyn, "Dallas Hospital Deals with Aftermath."

41. David Lauter, "Public Concerns about Ebola Increase Faster than Cases," *Los Angeles Times,* October 21, 2014, accessed October 23, 2014, http://www.latimes.com/nation/la-na-ebola-polls-20141021-story.html.

42. Ibid.

43. Eric Aasen and Krystina Martinez, "Dallas County tells 75 Presbyterian Workers to Stay Home," KERA News, Dallas, October 16, 2014, http://keranews.org/post/dallas-county-tells-75-presbyterian-workers-stay-home.

44. Lindsey Bever, "Chain Reaction: Concern about Ebola Nurse's Flight Prompts School Closings in Two States," *Washington Post,* October 16, 2014, http://www.washingtonpost.com/news/morning-mix/wp/2014/10/16/after-concern-about-ebola-patients-flight-schools-close-in-two-cities/.

45. Anica Padilla, "Two Frontier Airlines Planes that Carried Latest Ebola Patient at DIA for Extensive Cleaning." ABC 7 News, Denver, October 16, 2014, http://www.thedenverchannel.com/news/local-news/2-frontier-airlines-planes-that-carried-latest-ebola-patient-at-dia-for-extensive-cleaning.

46. Sydney Lupkin, "Ebola Scare Turns Dallas Hospital into a 'Ghost Town,'" ABC News, October 18, 2014, accessed January 4, 2015, http://abcnews.go.com/Health/ebola-scare-turns-dallas-hospital-ghost-town/story?id=26276610.

47. Sack, "Downfall for Hospital where Ebola Spread."

48. Liz Szabo, "Nurses Group Slams Dallas Hospital for Sloppy Ebola Care," *USA Today,* October 16, 2014, http://www.usatoday.com/story/news/nation/2014/10/15/nurses-protest-ebola/17302987/.

49. Goodwyn, "Dallas Hospital Deals with Aftermath."

50. St. Louis, "Hospitals in the U.S. Get Ready for Ebola."

51. Goodwyn, "Dallas Hospital Deals with Aftermath."

52. Sack, "Downfall for Hospital where Ebola Spread."

53. Fernandez and Healy, "C.D.C. Says it Should Have Responded Faster."

54. Fernandez and Sack, "Ebola Patient Sent Home Despite Fever, Records Show"; Seema Yasmin and Kimberly Railey, "Texas Health Presbyterian Begins Public Relations Effort to Restore Trust," *Dallas Morning News,* October 17, 2014, http://www.dallasnews.com/news/metro/20141017-presbyterian-begins-public-relations-effort-to-restore-trust.ece.

55. Anna Driver, "Texas Hospital Aims to Restore Image after Ebola Infections," Reuters, October 17, 2014, http://www.reuters.com/article/2014/10/17/us-health-ebola-usa-dallas-idUSKCN0I62AO20141017.

56. Fraser Seitel, "Rebuilding a Reputation Scorched by Ebola," *Forbes*, October 20, 2014, http://www.forbes.com/sites/fraserseitel/2014/10/20/rebuilding-a-reputation-scorched-by-ebola/.

57. Yasmin and Railey, "Texas Health Presbyterian Begins Public Relations Effort."

58. US House Energy and Commerce Committee, Subcommittee on Oversight and Investigations, Testimony of Dr. Daniel Varga, October 16, 2014, http://docs.house.gov/meetings/IF/IF02/20141016/102718/HHRG-113-IF02-Wstate-VargaD-20141016.pdf.

59. Jon Swaine, "Texas Hospital Mounts '#PresbyProud' Fightback as Ebola Criticism Mounts," *The Guardian*, October 18, 2014, http://www.theguardian.com/world/2014/oct/18/texas-ebola-hospital-presbyproud-fightback-criticism.

60. Sydney Lupkin, "Former President George W. Bush Visits Dallas Hospital that Faced Ebola," ABC News, November 7, 2014, http://abcnews.go.com/Health/president-george-bush-visits-dallas-hospital-faced-ebola/story?id=26764282.

61. Swaine, "Texas Hospital Mounts '#PresbyProud' Fightback."

62. Peter S. Goodman, "In Case of Emergency: What Not to Do," *The New York Times*, August 21, 2010, http://www.nytimes.com/2010/08/22/business/22crisis.html?pagewanted=all.

63. Peter M. Sandman, "How to Reassure Without Over-Reassuring," handout from Crisis Communication: Guidelines for Action, a DVD produced by the American Industrial Hygiene Association, May 2004, http://www.psandman.com/handouts/AIHA-DVD.htm.

64. "Calm Down America, Ebola Isn't about to Kill Us All," *Los Angeles Times*, editorial, October 20, 2014, http://www.latimes.com/opinion/editorials/la-ed-1021-ebola-panic-20141021-story.html.

65. Sandman, "How to Reassure Without Over-Reassuring."

66. "In U.S., an Ebola Crisis of Confidence," *Los Angeles Times*, editorial, October 15, 2014, http://www.latimes.com/opinion/editorials/la-ed-ebola-20141016-story.html.

67. "Four Lessons from Ebola Wars: Our View," *USA Today*, editorial, June 9, 2015, http://www.usatoday.com/story/opinion/2015/06/09/ebola-world-health-organization-g7-cdc-editorials-debates/28759663/.

68. Sandman, "How to Reassure Without Over-Reassuring."

69. Ibid.

70. William L. Benoit, "Image Repair Discourse and Crisis Communication," *Public Relations Review* 23, no. 2 (1997).

71. Jeffrey Weiss, "Dallas-Area Officials, Health Experts Discuss Lessons of Recent Ebola Crisis," *Dallas Morning News*, November 5, 2104, http://www.dallasnews.com/ebola/headlines/20141105-dallas-area-officials-health-experts-discuss-lessons-of-recent-ebola-crisis.ece.

72. Vincent T. Covello, "Risk and Crisis Communication: Communicating Effectively in High Concern, High Stress, or Low Trust Situations," presentation to California Department of Public Health, n.d., accessed July 23, 2015, http://www.cdph.ca.gov/programs/cobbh/Documents/10%20DR.%20VINCENT%20COVELLO%20a.Slides.San%20Diego.pdf.

73. Matthew Watkins, "Dallas County Judge Clay Jenkins' High Profile Attracts Praise, Scorn," *Dallas Morning News*, October 9, 2014, http://www.dallasnews.com/news/metro/20141009-dallas-county-judge-clay-jenkins-high-profile-attracts-praise-scorn.ece.

74. Manny Fernandez, "Dallas Official Confronts City's Fear of Ebola in Person," *The New York Times*, October 10, 2014, http://www.nytimes.com/2014/10/11/us/ebola-dallas-clay-jenkins.html.

75. George Merlis, "Three Ways to Stop the Ebola Panic," *Fortune*, October 28, 2014, http://fortune.com/2014/10/28/ebola-panic-confidence/.

76. Mora and Dalrymple, "Can Texas Hospital Recover from Ebola Scare?"; Swaine, "Texas Hospital Mounts '#PresbyProud' Fightback."

77. Mora and Dalrymple, "Can Texas Hospital Recover from Ebola Scare?"

78. Seitel, "Rebuilding a Reputation Scorched by Ebola."

V Ethics and Ebola

13 The Use and Study of Unregistered Ebola Interventions: Ethics and Equipoise

Michael J. Selgelid

Use of Unregistered Interventions

The World Health Organization (WHO) declared the Ebola virus disease (EVD) outbreak in West Africa a public health emergency of international concern on August 8, 2014. At the time, 1,711 cases of EVD, and 932 deaths, had been reported.[1]

The following week, on August 11, 2014, WHO convened an advisory ethics panel "to consider and assess the ethical implications for clinical decision-making [regarding the] use of unregistered interventions [for EVD] that have shown promising results in the laboratory and in animal models but that have not yet been evaluated for safety and efficacy in humans."[2] This meeting was (presumably) largely motivated by high-profile (media) controversy surrounding treatment of health care workers from wealthy developed nations (that became infected with Ebola in West Africa) with the monoclonal antibody ZMapp upon return to their home countries. The use of ZMapp in such patients was controversial partly because it raised questions about why (only) health workers from wealthy developed countries were being treated with this intervention (in very short supply) rather than patients in West Africa. The use of ZMapp was also controversial because this intervention had never previously been tested or used in humans, whereas standard medical practice is that the earliest human use of an intervention generally occurs in Phase 1 clinical trials—for evaluation of safety—prior to actual use in patients.

The WHO panel was thus posed with the question whether it is ethically acceptable to use unregistered medications that have never previously been tested in humans in the context of the emergency Ebola crisis unfolding in West Africa. In addition to ZMapp, this question was relevant to numerous other candidate drugs and vaccines there was reason to believe might be promising interventions against Ebola, though they had likewise never been previously tested in humans. Some of these other interventions, like ZMapp, had shown especially promising results in animal studies.

In response to this question, the panel members unanimously concluded that it may be ethically acceptable to use unregistered medications (not previously tested in humans) in the context of the emergency EVD situation, so long as various basic ethical conditions are met:

The ethical criteria include transparency about all aspects of care, so that maximum information is obtained about the effects of the interventions, fair distribution in the face of scarcity, promotion of cosmopolitan solidarity, informed consent, freedom of choice, confidentiality, respect for the person, preservation of dignity and involvement of the community. Use of these interventions should also be based on the best possible assessment of risk and benefit from the available information.[3]

The panel furthermore concluded that when interventions are used in such contexts, it is important that we learn as much as possible about the safety and efficacy of the interventions in question:

if and when these interventions are used to treat patients (or as prevention), the physicians overseeing their administration have a moral obligation to collect and share all scientifically relevant data generated, including from treatment provided for "compassionate use" (access to an unapproved drug outside a clinical trial), in order to establish the safety and efficacy of the interventions.

The group discussed how use of these investigational interventions in a clinical context can be evaluated scientifically to ensure timely, accurate information about their safety and efficacy. They agreed unanimously that investigators have a moral duty to evaluate these interventions (for treatment or prevention) in the best possible clinical studies that can be conducted under the circumstances of the epidemic in order to establish their safety and efficacy or to provide evidence to stop their use. Continuous evaluation should guide future interventions.[4]

This insistence on scientific evaluation of the use of unregistered interventions is at least partly justifiable on justice grounds. The fact that there were not already registered interventions against Ebola, that is, arguably reflected prior wrongs. Given familiarity with Ebola for almost forty years before the West African outbreak, one might have expected that there should already have been more testing and development of interventions against the disease—and that we should not, in 2014, have been in a situation where it was necessary to resort to the use of unregistered medications that had not yet even gone through Phase 1 trials in the first place. Why were there not already registered interventions against Ebola, and why were we not already further down the research and development pipeline for Ebola vaccines and therapeutics? One reason more Ebola countermeasure research and development had not already previously taken place is presumably that we rely so heavily upon private enterprise—that is, pharmaceutical companies with profit-driven, self-interested motives—to determine what research does and does not get done. The previous 40 years of experience with Ebola was limited to small outbreaks in rural villages in poor African countries. Given that it had previously only affected small numbers of people in poor countries, Ebola was not the kind of disease that would appear to provide good return on investment—and so the lack of more Ebola countermeasure research and development is ultimately unsurprising. One lesson learned from the Ebola epidemic is arguably that it is a mistake to rely so heavily on private enterprise to develop and provide solutions to what are ultimately public problems.

Equipoise and Prioritization of Use and Study of Unregistered Interventions

The WHO panel's insistence on scientific evaluation of the use of unregistered interventions, in any case, raised further questions about the ethics of scientifically studying the use of such interventions in the emergency context of Ebola. Regarding the question of who should be prioritized to receive experimental interventions in limited supply or where relevant studies should take place, the WHO Ebola Ethics Working Group (tasked with addressing this and related questions) ultimately concluded:

> The recipients of experimental interventions, locations of studies, and study design should be based on the aim to learn as much as possible, as quickly as possible, without compromising patient care, local community values or health worker safety. Trials should be designed and conducted with the active participation of local scientists and researchers, and with proper consultation with communities and local ethics committees.[5]

It is noteworthy that this answer differs from those commonly given to questions about who should be prioritized to receive limited supplies of drugs, vaccines, and so on in other contexts. In the context of pandemic influenza, for example, it has commonly been argued that health care workers and children should be prioritized to receive interventions in limited supply in order to promote both utility and fairness.[6] A utilitarian reason to prioritize health workers is that health workers are needed to fight pandemics—so keeping health workers healthy and alive has especially important societal benefits. A fairness-based reason appeals to the principle of reciprocity: Health workers provide a valuable service to humanity by facing risks associated with health care provision, so society owes them something back in return. A utilitarian reason for prioritizing children over older persons is that, other things being equal, more lost years of life can be averted by saving the life of a younger rather than an older person. A fairness-based argument for prioritizing children appeals to the "fair innings" argument—the idea being that it would be unfair if a child is killed prematurely and thus does not have the opportunity to live through all the stages of life (which, according to some, one has a right to do).

Both kinds of rationales in both kinds of cases, however, depend on the presumption that we are talking about prioritization of interventions that are safe and effective, and ultimately expected to be beneficial. This, however, cannot be taken for granted in the context of unregistered, experimental interventions that have not previously been tested in humans. Whether or not such rationales for resolving questions regarding resource allocation in pandemics should also apply to questions surrounding prioritization of unregistered experimental Ebola interventions depends on whether there is reason to be confident that recipients of such interventions are more likely than not to benefit from the interventions in question. Even in cases where there have been especially promising (safety and efficacy) results in animal testing of an intervention, this may not provide grounds for confidence that the intervention in question would be beneficial to humans—because it is notoriously difficult to translate animal findings to humans. Whether there were good grounds for confidence that particular candidate Ebola interventions would have been more likely than not to benefit human recipients is ultimately a scientific question beyond the scope of this chapter. The main point for now, in any case, is that answers to ethical questions about prioritization of unregistered Ebola interventions ultimately depend on answers to this kind of scientific question (which has not, to my knowledge,[7] been answered).

While the above rationales for prioritization of limited interventions (proven to be safe and effective) in pandemics may not help answer questions about who should be prioritized to receive experimental interventions for which we are in a state of equipoise—that is, where there is no reason to be confident that the intervention is likely to be more beneficial than available alternatives, or vice versa—there may still be good reasons to prioritize health workers in the latter kind of case. In light of the WHO Ebola Ethics Working Group's statement that prioritization decisions should, inter alia, "be based on the aim to learn as much as possible, as quickly as possible," a reason to prioritize health workers, at least in the case of vaccine trials, is that (other things being equal) it is possible to learn more about the efficacy of a vaccine by using it in those most likely to be exposed to the pathogen in question; and health care workers treating Ebola patients are especially likely to be exposed to the Ebola virus. Another good reason for prioritizing health care workers is that they are more likely to be able to give proper informed consent, especially in the West African countries most heavily impacted by Ebola—because health workers are among the most literate citizens of these countries (and because they have specialized knowledge especially apt for informed consent to medical intervention).

Equipoise and Placebo-Controlled Trials

The question of equipoise is likewise relevant to questions surrounding the ethical design of scientific studies of unregistered Ebola interventions. While some have voiced opposition to placebo-controlled trials of Ebola therapeutics because this would deprive some patient-participants (i.e., those who end up receiving placebo) with a highly fatal disease from potentially efficacious therapy[8]—the idea that it would be unfortunate to receive placebo rather than the intervention being tested depends on the presumption that there is reason to be confident the intervention being tested is actually more beneficial than placebo. If (despite promising results in animals) we really are in a state of equipoise, then there is no reason to believe it would be worse to receive placebo than the intervention under investigation. In addition to uncertainty about efficacy, uncertainty about safety of unregistered experimental interventions would remain even after Phase 1 trials are conducted—so receipt of an experimental intervention could do more harm than good (i.e., it might ultimately be preferable to receive placebo rather than the experimental intervention). Those who receive placebo in such a trial, in any case, would not be deprived of anything available to those who do not, or are unable, to participate in trials to begin with (which would inevitably be the case for many Ebola patients given limited supply of numerous candidate experimental Ebola interventions)—so (other things being equal) no harm would result from participation in a placebo-controlled trial. If it is assumed for the sake of argument that the intervention under investigation is likely to be more beneficial than placebo, on the other hand, then one would arguably benefit from participation in a placebo-controlled trial—because one could thus gain the opportunity (not available to nonparticipants) to receive the intervention.[9] One of the main objections to placebo-controlled trials of Ebola therapeutics (i.e., that such trials would deprive participants of access to potentially beneficial interventions) is thus arguably unpersuasive whether or not there is a state of equipoise.

A better reason for being ethically opposed to conducting placebo-controlled trials of Ebola interventions in the most heavily affected countries, on the other hand, is that representatives of these countries repeatedly made clear at WHO meetings that local communities would consider such trials to be unacceptable (precisely because of perception that such trials would deprive some participants of access to potentially beneficial interventions). Whether or not more or better community engagement (e.g., explaining the usual rational for placebo-controlled trials and why there might not be any good reason to assume that those who receive placebo would be disadvantaged if there really is a state of equipoise) would have changed local community attitudes toward, or resulted in acceptance of, placebo-controlled trials is perhaps an open question. Effective community engagement regarding such matters in the context of the Ebola crisis in West Africa, however, might not have been very easy given the actual situation on the ground.[10] Whether or not local community rejection of placebo-controlled trials is ultimately rational or well-informed, local community acceptance is arguably a necessary condition of the ethical acceptability of research involving human subjects.[11]

Acknowledgment

Though I was a member of the WHO ethics panel and WHO working group discussed in this chapter, opinions expressed here are my own rather than (except where explicitly stated) those of WHO.

Notes

1. World Health Organization, "Statement of the 1st Meeting of the IHR Emergency Committee on the 2014 Ebola Outbreak in West Africa," 2014, http://www.who.int/mediacentre/news/statements/2014/ebola-20140808/en/.

2. World Health Organization, "Ethical Considerations for Use of Unregistered Interventions for Ebola Virus Disease: Report of an Advisory Panel," 2014, http://apps.who.int/iris/bitstream/10665/130997/1/WHO_HIS_KER_GHE_14.1_eng.pdf?ua=1.

3. Ibid.

4. Ibid.

5. World Health Organization, 2014, "Ethical Issues Related to Study Design for Trials on Therapeutics for Ebola Virus Disease," http://apps.who.int/iris/bitstream/10665/137509/1/WHO_HIS_KER_GHE_14.2_eng.pdf?ua=1.

6. M. J. Selgelid, "Pandethics," *Public Health*, 123, no. 3 (2009): 255–59.

7. Despite participation in numerous relevant meetings where this kind of question was asked.

8. C. Adebamowo, O. Bah-Sow, F. Binka, R. Bruzzone, A. Caplan, J. F. Delfraissy, et al., "Randomized Controlled Trials for Ebola: Practical and Ethical Issues," *Lancet*, 384, no. 9952 (2014): 1423–24.

9. J. Cohen, "Issues continue to dog the testing of Ebola drugs and vaccines," *Science*, October 16, 2014, http://news.sciencemag.org/health/2014/10/issues-continue-dog-testing-ebola-drugs-and-vaccines.

10. As Ebola health worker colleagues have noted. "How," they asked, "would you go about it?"

11. World Health Organization, "Ethical Issues Related to Study Design for Trials on Therapeutics for Ebola Virus Disease," 2014. http://apps.who.int/iris/bitstream/10665/137509/1/WHO_HIS_KER_GHE_14.2_eng.pdf?ua=1.

14 (How) Should Experimental Vaccines and Treatments for Ebola Be Used?

Annette Rid

Background

In 2013, the world began to witness an unprecedented Ebola epidemic in West Africa that is now smoldering. Weak health systems were primarily to blame for the resulting suffering and loss of life. A few years earlier, one of the discoverers of the Ebola virus said that Ebola is "really a disease of poverty and neglect of health systems."[1] With adequate health systems and basic infrastructure in place, the epidemic would likely have been contained in its early stages.

Absent such systems and infrastructure, the outbreak quickly seemed to spiral out of control. In August 2014, the World Health Organization (WHO) declared the epidemic a public health emergency of international concern, which is a formal declaration of a public health crisis with potentially global reach under international health regulations.[2] Clinical trials of experimental Ebola vaccines and treatments soon emerged as a key component of the global response. These experimental interventions were in the earliest phases of testing at the beginning of the outbreak, and whether and how they should be used caused heated controversy, not only among investigators, sponsors, and host communities, but also among bioethicists.

This chapter offers an overview of the ethical debate about the use of experimental Ebola interventions during the ongoing outbreak. It first describes four major challenges for using unproven vaccines and treatments during this epidemic. It then discusses whether it is ethical to conduct trials given these challenges and, if so, under which conditions experimental interventions should be tested. Reflecting the debate up to

July 2015, when this chapter was written, issues around trial design receive special attention.

Four Challenges for Using Experimental Interventions in the Ongoing Ebola Epidemic

As concern about the Ebola outbreak waxed in 2014, four major challenges emerged around using the available unproven treatments and vaccines. The first challenge was an acute sense of *urgency* to deploy the experimental interventions and, some argued, get trials off the ground. Previous Ebola outbreaks had fatality rates as high as 90 percent, and, to date, there were no proven vaccines or specific treatments for the disease.[3] Many cautioned that experimental interventions were unlikely to make an impact on this epidemic, but the possibility that a "magic bullet" might be among these interventions remained a powerful motive for endorsing their use. When some experts warned that more than a million people in Liberia and Sierra Leone could be infected with Ebola by early 2015,[4] and there were concerns that the disease might become endemic in the region or spread globally,[5] the use of potentially effective vaccines and specific treatments seemed more pressing still.

The second challenge was profound *uncertainty* about both Ebola virus disease and the existing experimental vaccines and treatments for the disease. Before this outbreak, Ebola had claimed less than 3,000 lives cumulatively over four decades. Previous epidemics had occurred in rural areas and had been relatively easy to contain, involving at most 500 patients per outbreak.[6] Given this, insight into the natural progression of Ebola and its prevention or treatment was extremely limited before this epidemic.[7] In addition, several unique features emerged during this epidemic that increased uncertainty about whether the Ebola virus had been, or was, evolving. Specifically, the outbreak occurred for the first time in urban areas, and it spread exponentially for several months, leading to fears that dangerous viral mutations might occur.

Because the burden of disease from Ebola virus was limited before this outbreak, research on Ebola was limited as well. Some governments of high-income countries funded research into vaccines and specific treatments because they feared the Ebola virus might be used as a biological weapon, given the high fatality rate of the disease.[8] This research had identified several interventions; however, all of them were in the earliest phases of testing when this epidemic broke. For example, ZMapp—a combination of monoclonal antibodies—was under study in primates when it was first administered to two US citizens who had contracted Ebola in July 2014 in Liberia.[9]

Other potential specific therapies for Ebola were just as poorly understood. A number of investigational or licensed interventions targeted at diseases other than Ebola were being explored for their anti-Ebola activity, but clinical testing was far into the future.[10] In addition, no more than a few Ebola patients had ever received blood or plasma from survivors prior to 2014. The uncertainty around Ebola virus disease was therefore compounded by a profound uncertainty about the existing experimental interventions for Ebola.

Major *feasibility constraints* were the third challenge in providing clinical care and preventive services or conducting clinical research. The epidemic occurred in some of the least-developed countries[11] and brought weak health systems to a near-complete collapse, deepened distrust of health providers within the population, and even resulted in aggression against a small number of them. Moreover, preexisting research capacity and infrastructure were extremely limited in the affected region, and historical cases of abuse and misconduct by researchers from high-income countries loomed over research efforts during this epidemic.[12]

The fourth challenge was deep *ethical controversy* about how the experimental interventions should be used in light of the above considerations. This is the topic of the remainder of this chapter.

Are Clinical Trials of Experimental Ebola Interventions Ethical?

Two fundamental questions quickly dominated the debate. First, should the existing experimental vaccines and treatments for Ebola be used? Second, if the answer were yes, should they be deployed as part of clinical trials or as part of what might be called "experimental clinical care or prevention," or—more conventionally—"compassionate use"? These questions were precipitated by the use of ZMapp and other experimental interventions, such as whole blood transfusion, when several health care workers from high-income countries were infected with Ebola.[13] The WHO took a leading role in the ensuing debate and convened an international panel that endorsed the use of unproven vaccines and treatments provided a range of ethical criteria were met.[14]

Should Experimental Vaccines and Treatments Be Used?

The WHO recommendation was appropriate for several reasons. Even with effective supportive treatment—fluid replacement, broad-spectrum antibiotics, malaria treatment, and antipyretics—it was considered unlikely that fatality rates could be lowered to below 30 percent.[15] Moreover, when the WHO made its recommendation, the fatality from Ebola was estimated to be at 50–70 percent because patients were diagnosed late and treatment centers were overrun.[16] Given these grim prospects, it was reasonable to ask patients to assume considerable risks from early experimental interventions—or, more precisely, considerable uncertainty about their risks and potential benefits—in order to potentially save their lives or contribute to curbing a dangerous epidemic.

The argument for the use of the available experimental interventions is weaker for vaccines than for treatments because healthy individuals have alternative means of preventing an infection, such as wearing personal protective equipment and practicing good hygiene. However, investigational vaccines against serious diseases like Ebola tend to pose lower risks than investigational treatments for these diseases, given that vaccines are administered to healthy individuals and therefore expected to be much safer than treatments for patients whose lives are at risk. Moreover, as the high number of infected health workers in this epidemic illustrates,[17] some populations have an increased risk of contracting Ebola virus disease due to higher exposure to the virus or inadequate protections (or both). Greater risks from early experimental vaccines thus seem reasonable as well, especially in health workers, burial teams, and other at-risk populations.

Furthermore, testing the existing unproven interventions is critical for an effective response to large-scale epidemics in the future, and robust data can only be collected when sufficiently large numbers of individuals are affected (i.e., during an outbreak). Given that Ebola virus strikes unpredictably, and—before this outbreak—typically affected small numbers of people, there may not be an opportunity to pursue larger trials in the near future. The fact that evaluating the experimental interventions has important social value in helping to potentially control a virulent infectious disease, and that there are few alternatives to gathering data during an epidemic, further supports the reasonableness of accepting increased levels of risk or uncertainty.

Some also argued that using the experimental interventions could be instrumental for curbing the ongoing epidemic, notably by providing infected individuals with an incentive to seek care, potentially identifying a "game-changing" vaccine or treatment for Ebola and promoting public trust.[18] Such arguments for the use of experimental interventions should be treated with caution. All of them build on the hope that the investigational vaccines and treatments will make at-risk populations and patients better off, or at least not worse off. However, under ordinary circumstances, only 10 percent of investigational agents beginning phase 1 make it to commercial launch,[19] and some cause serious harms that were unpredictable at the start. This percentage may have been even lower for the existing Ebola interventions, given the limited clinical and preclinical data on their effects. More realism about the effects of unproven agents is warranted, even if this can be psychologically difficult when a deadly outbreak is seemingly spiraling out of control.

Instrumental arguments for the use of experimental interventions also assume that such use will not compromise the general response to the epidemic. However, there are several ways in which the use of experimental interventions might compromise containment and care. For example, public trust can be undermined, notably when unproven agents prove harmful or, in the case of clinical trials, communities in need do not receive fair benefits from the research.[20] For instance, complex treatments like ZMapp—which is expensive to produce and requires intravenous administration—are unlikely to be implemented in resource-poor settings in the near future, and trust could be undermined if communities do not obtain access to any proven, effective interventions from the research. Experimental vaccines can also complicate containment if they cause Ebola-like symptoms and thereby put further pressure on health systems. These issues are obviously complex and require more research. Yet the above examples suggest that the use of experimental interventions can have a negative impact on the general outbreak response, so that priorities between such use and containment or care may need to be set.

Importantly, the WHO did not adequately address this issue. It stated, "investigational therapeutic or prophylactic options should not divert attention or resources from the public health measures that remain the main priority in outbreak control."[21] Yet this position ignores potentially unavoidable conflicts between using investigational vaccines and treatments and efforts to contain the epidemic or care for patients, especially in the context of weak or collapsing health systems. More generally, the WHO seemed to have no clear strategy for how to integrate the use of experimental interventions into the general response to the outbreak. The organization declared the epidemic a public health emergency of international concern on August 8, 2014, and published a short web summary of its recommendation to use the existing experimental interventions just four days later; this was more than two weeks before its general "Ebola Response Roadmap" was completed.[22] Despite the urgency of the situation, a clearer and more realistic vision for how to integrate the use of unproven vaccines or treatments and the broader outbreak response would have been helpful—especially since the WHO was poised to take the international lead for coordinating trials or experimental care or prevention.[23, 24]

Should Experimental Interventions Be Used in Trials or as Part of Clinical Care or Prevention?

While there was broad agreement that it was acceptable to use the available unproven vaccines and treatments, controversy arose as to whether they should be deployed in clinical trials or as part of (monitored) experimental clinical care or prevention. The difference between the two can be more or less pronounced depending on the trial design. Individually randomized, controlled trials (IRCTs) include a control group that does not receive the investigational vaccine or treatment. This is a stark contrast to experimental clinical care or prevention, where all individuals or patients are eligible to receive the investigational agent, barring limitations in supply and countervailing clinical judgment. Uncontrolled trials fall between these two poles because they specify conditions for providing the experimental agents—for example, eligibility criteria and stopping rules—while still providing everyone who qualifies with an investigational vaccine or treatment. Data on patient outcomes are gathered in clinical trials as well as experimental clinical care and prevention, although the data collection is more limited in the latter.

The question of whether trials or experimental care and prevention were appropriate opened deep rifts about the norms that should guide the use of existing experimental interventions during this outbreak. Those who took a clinical perspective argued for experimental clinical care and prevention, trying to do everything possible for individuals who currently suffer from a life-threatening disease or are at risk of contracting it. By contrast, those who took a research perspective argued for clinical trials that enhance potential benefits for individual participants to the extent this is compatible with generating valid data for the benefit of future populations. The disagreement is apparent in the WHO statement that "compassionate use is justified as an exceptional emergency measure"; it remains unclear whether the Ebola outbreak as a whole qualifies as an emergency that justifies compassionate use, or whether the term emergency is more confined.[25] Conversely, some commentators have argued that experimental clinical care or prevention is a "serious mistake" and should be avoided.[26] While these claims were made early in the debate and might therefore lack nuance, they illustrate the deep disagreement about whether a clinical or a research perspective on the existing experimental interventions should be adopted.

A more balanced position points to considerations that support trials in some cases and emergency clinical care or prevention in others.[27] For example, if an experimental intervention is promising based on preclinical or clinical data, and known to be safe, plentiful, and easy to administer, it might be offered to all patients outside of formal trials. Imagine that evidence suggests a daily vitamin C pill could improve clinical outcomes in Ebola patients. Experimental clinical care could be justified in this case because patients are unlikely to experience harm, vitamin C is readily available, and the costs of providing it—with respect to production, supply, and clinical administration—are low.[28] By contrast, if an experimental intervention is scarce or costly and its safety uncertain, trials seem more appropriate so that it can be evaluated more systematically and the available stocks are used to this effect. Nonetheless, how these and other considerations are weighed critically depends on whether one believes that clinical or research norms should guide the use of experimental interventions, and how these norms should be specified in a situation of crisis. More analysis of these issues, notably the latter question, is needed.

Overall, the above considerations suggest that clinical trials were generally more appropriate in the ongoing epidemic than experimental care or prevention. Most investigational vaccines and treatments were neither known to be safe nor widely available, and their clinical benefits were highly uncertain. Many agents were also costly to produce or complex to administer. This suggests that trials of the experimental interventions were generally preferable, not only to avoid harm to healthy individuals or patients, but also to determine whether producing and deploying these interventions on a larger scale would be a reasonable investment.

Under Which Conditions Are Clinical Trials of Experimental Ebola Interventions Ethical?

Once it has been determined that an experimental intervention should be evaluated in a trial, it is important to determine how recognized ethical criteria for research—such as a reasonable risk-benefit ratio, fair participant selection, and informed consent—should be applied given the particular challenges of this epidemic.[29] The criteria had some reasonably straightforward implications.[30] For example, the informed consent criterion requires that information be disclosed, and that voluntary and informed consent be obtained, in culturally and linguistically appropriate formats. The criterion of independent review requires that public accountability regarding the trials be ensured through ethical oversight and review. However, other implications were less straightforward (see table 14.1).

For instance, how should speed and rigor be balanced in research ethics review? What should determine the selection of trial sites so as to meet the criterion of fair participant selection? Who should be prioritized for trial enrollment? A growing literature has been addressing these issues,[31] often building on prior work on the ethics of conducting research during epidemics and other disasters.[32]

The remainder of this section explores the question that has dominated the ethical debate so far, namely whether trials should be conducted using individually randomized, controlled or uncontrolled designs. This question has polarized commentators, with some advocating IRCTs[33] and others rejecting them on both ethical and practical grounds.[34] The question also divided a subsequent WHO Ethics Working Group on treatment trials; some members of the group considered IRCTs unethical in certain situations, while others regarded trials without a control group equally unethical if the trial design led to uninterpretable or misleading results.[35] The fundamental issue at stake is whether investigators are required to provide the experimental vaccine or treatment under study to *all* trial participants. If the answer is yes, then an IRCT that randomizes a control group to standard prevention or supportive care without providing the experimental intervention—or providing the intervention at a later point in time—is ethically unacceptable.

The debate was particularly heated in the context of treatment trials, compared to vaccine trials, and will be the focus here. It primarily revolved around three of the recognized ethical criteria for research.[36] First, the criterion of a reasonable risk-benefit ratio requires that the risks which research interventions pose to participants be reasonable in relation to the potential clinical benefits for them; the scientific and social value of the research; or both.[37] Whether risks and potential benefits are reasonable from the individual participants' perspective depends, among other things, on their available alternatives for treatment. Some commentators have argued that the outcomes of supportive care—the only available treatment during this epidemic—were so poor that the risk-benefit ratio for participants would be reasonable only when all received the study intervention.[38] However, although fatality rates with supportive care varied considerably between locations and over time, they were as low as 30 percent in some treatment centers.[39] Moreover, some humanitarian aid organizations argued that more aggressive care could decrease fatality from Ebola to 10 percent.[40] If one considers these numbers together with the often profound uncertainty about the unproven treatments, including their potential to harm individuals who battle a life-threatening disease, participants' interest in receiving an investigational agent looks much less compelling. While these risk-benefit judgments will ultimately depend on the specific treatment under study as well as the outcomes of locally feasible supportive care, it appears that receiving supportive care in the control group was not a clearly unreasonable option for participants in at least some treatment trials.

Second, there are other ethical criteria that interact with risk-benefit considerations for individual participants, notably the criterion of scientific validity. This criterion reflects investigators' fundamental obligation to conduct socially valuable and scientifically sound research; when a study

Table 14.1
Ethical issues regarding the conduct of clinical trials in the ongoing Ebola outbreak

Ethical criteria	Key issues
Collaborative partnership	• How can meaningful community engagement in the planning, conduct, and oversight of trials be achieved in a time of crisis? • How can fair benefits from the conduct or results of trials be ensured (e.g., contribute to containment efforts, help to ensure availability of any proven effective vaccines or treatments)? • How can collaboration between trial partners be promoted (e.g., academic and private sponsors, humanitarian aid organizations)? • How can responsibilities be shared fairly among trial partners (e.g., trial insurance)?
Social value	• Which experimental interventions should be prioritized for study? Based on which criteria (e.g., expected safety or efficacy, availability, cost)? • How much priority should generally be given to research on diseases with catastrophic potential (e.g., emerging infectious diseases like Ebola)? • When does research unduly compromise efforts to contain the epidemic or treat affected patients?
Scientific validity	• What level of evidence about the experimental interventions is needed to inform decisions about the need for additional research, marketing approval or withdrawal, or large-scale implementation? • Which trial design(s) are likely to produce this evidence? • To what extent should practical constraints such as infrastructure and staffing determine trial design? • To what extent should concerns about public trust determine trial design?
Fair selection of study participants and populations	• Which criteria should determine the selection of trial sites (e.g., ability to benefit participants or meet recruitment targets)? • When should trial sites be closed? Based on which criteria? • Who should be prioritized for trial enrolment? Based on which criteria (e.g., reciprocity, utility, ability to consent, ability to meet the scientific goals of the trial)? • How can adherence to specified eligibility criteria be ensured in practice? • Does the enrolment of families require special consideration? • What are appropriate safeguards for enrolling especially vulnerable groups (e.g., orphans, pregnant women)?

Table 14.1 (continued)

Ethical criteria	Key issues
Acceptable risk-benefit ratio	• When are experimental interventions promising enough for clinical trials? Based on what kind of data? • Is it acceptable to withhold experimental interventions from a control group? If so, under which conditions? • How should the requirements to reduce risks and enhance potential benefits for participants be balanced with each other, as well as with potentially competing considerations, such as fair participant selection and scientific validity? • When is the risk-benefit ratio for research staff acceptable (e.g., research procedures that expose staff to risks)?
Independent review	• How should speed and rigor be balanced in ethical review and oversight (e.g., expedited review vs. review by full committee)? • What should happen if no local or national ethical review committee is in place?
Informed consent	• How can informed consent or surrogate consent be obtained in a situation of crisis? • What should be done if a surrogate decision maker for incapacitated patients is not available (e.g., independent patient advocate)? • When are supplementary community or familial consent procedures appropriate?
Respect for recruited study participants and communities	• How can the confidentiality of recruited or enrolled participants be ensured under the complex conditions of an epidemic? • What level of ancillary care are participants owed in a situation of crisis? • What are researchers and sponsors' obligations to participants after the trial is completed (e.g., transition to care after research, follow-up research)?

Note: Because reasonable people will disagree about many of these issues, fair and accountable procedures for making respective decisions are essential. The ethical criteria are adapted from the work by Emanuel and colleagues.[26]

fails to address an important question by using adequate methods, it is widely considered to be ethically unacceptable.[41] However, the obligation to conduct valid research is constrained by investigators' duty to reduce and limit risks to those that are reasonable in relation to the potential social value of the research, as well as the duty to enhance potential benefits for participants.[42]

Under ordinary circumstances, these two duties are not equivalent in moral force. Investigators' negative duty to limit excessive risks acts as a strong constraint on conducting valid research, implying that studies should not be conducted if the risks are unacceptable. By contrast, investigators' positive duty to benefit participants is much weaker, and it is constrained to the extent that enhancing potential benefits to participants is consistent with designs that produce valid data to socially valuable questions.

The question is whether a public health crisis like the ongoing epidemic changes the relationship between investigators' duty to enhance benefits to participants and their obligation to conduct valid research. This question is still open and compounded by methodological controversy around the quality of the data that different trial designs are likely to yield under complex conditions like this epidemic. However, once it has been determined that an experimental treatment is not appropriate for emergency clinical care and should instead be evaluated in research, it is difficult to see how the duty to enhance potential benefits for participants could be so strong as to undermine the scientific validity of trials.

Third, in addition to scientific validity, the criterion of fair participant selection is likely to interact with risk-benefit considerations for individual participants.[43] Many of the experimental treatments for Ebola were in short supply because manufacturing capacity was limited, and public and private sponsors were reluctant to finance large-scale production based on limited data about the treatments' effects. This implies that not every patient who might benefit from the existing experimental interventions could receive access. More analysis of how fairness considerations affect the choice of trial design is needed. Yet it is possible that IRCTs—which are effectively a lottery—offer the fairest way of distributing investigational treatments under conditions of scarcity.[44]

Conclusion

Urgency, uncertainty, feasibility constraints, and ethical controversy likely pose challenges for all research that is being conducted during infectious outbreaks. However, the ongoing Ebola virus epidemic involved a unique constellation of these factors as very early experimental vaccines and treatments were being deployed in a rapidly evolving situation. The debate about whether and how to use these interventions was often polarized and did not pay sufficient attention to the complexity of the situation. The response to future epidemics will hopefully benefit from emerging insights into the numerous factors that influence the ethical use of experimental interventions under similar circumstances.

Acknowledgments

Many thanks to the editors of this volume—Nicholas Evans, Maimuna Majumder, and Tara Smith—and Franklin Miller and David Wendler for their very helpful comments on an earlier version of this chapter. Thanks also go to other colleagues who have influenced my views on this topic, in particular Ezekiel Emanuel, Steven Joffe, and Verina Wild, and to Rose Mortimer for help with formatting. The work benefited from a Caroline Miles Visiting Scholarship at the ETHOX Centre, University of Oxford, and was funded by the People Programme (Marie Curie Actions) of the European Union's Seventh Framework Programme (FP7/2007–2013) under REA grant agreement number 301816.

Notes

1. Peter Piot, *No Time to Lose: A Life in Pursuit of Deadly Viruses* (New York: W.W. Norton, 2012), 83.

2. World Health Organization, "WHO Statement on the Meeting of the International Health Regulations Emergency Committee Regarding the 2014 Ebola Outbreak in West Africa," August 8, 2014, http://www.who.int/mediacentre/news/statements/2014/ebola-20140808/en/. For more information on the International Health Regulations, please see Phelan's contribution in this volume, in chapter 9.

3. Heinz Feldmann and Thomas W. Geisbert, "Ebola Haemorrhagic Fever," *Lancet* 377, no. 9768 (2011): 849–62.

4. Martin I. Meltzer, Charisma Y. Atkins, Scott Santibanez, Barbara Knust, Brett W. Petersen, Elizabeth D. Ervin, et al., "Estimating the Future Number of Cases in the Ebola Epidemic—Liberia and Sierra Leone, 2014-2015," *Morbidity and Mortality Weekly Report* 63, no. 3 (September 2014): 1–14.

5. Maryn McKenna, "The grim future if Ebola goes global," *Wired*, October 27, 2014, http://www.wired.com/2014/10/ebola-endemic/.

6. Feldmann and Geisbert, "Ebola haemorrhagic fever."

7. Ibid.

8. Ibid.

9. Anthony S. Fauci, "Ebola—Underscoring the Global Disparities in Health Care Resources," *The New England Journal of Medicine* 371 (September 2014): 1084–6.

10. Martin Enserink, "Debate Erupts on 'Repurposed' Drugs for Ebola," *Science* 345, no. 6198 (2014): 718–19.

11. United Nations Development Programme, "Human Development Report 2014: Sustaining Human Progress: Reducing Vulnerabilities and Building Resilience," 2014, accessed 11 August, 2015, http://hdr.undp.org/sites/default/files/hdr14-report-en-1.pdf.

12. Jeanne Lenzer, "Secret Report Surfaces Showing That Pfizer Was at Fault in Nigerian Drug Tests," *British Medical Journal* 332, no. 7552 (2006): 1233.

13. Sophie Arie, "Ebola: An Opportunity for a Clinical Trial?" *BMJ* 349 (August 2014): g4997.

14. The panel listed the following ethical criteria, derived from "traditional research ethics, professional ethics, public health ethics and global health ethics": "transparency, … trust, fair distribution, … cosmopolitan solidarity, informed consent, freedom of choice, confidentiality, respect for the person, preservation of dignity, and involvement of the community." World Health Organization, "Ethical Considerations for Use of Unregistered Interventions for Ebola Viral Disease: Report of an Advisory Panel to WHO," 2014, accessed 6 July, 2015, www.who.int/csr/resources/publications/ebola/ethical-considerations/en/.

15. Feldmann and Geisbert, "Ebola haemorrhagic fever."

16. WHO Ebola Response Team, "Ebola Virus Disease in West Africa—The First 9 Months of the Epidemic and Forward Projections," *The New England Journal of Medicine* 371 (October 2014): 1481–95.

17. World Health Organization, "Health Worker Ebola Infections in Guinea, Liberia and Sierra Leone," 2015, accessed 12 August, 2015, http://apps.who.int/iris/bitstream/10665/171823/1/WHO_EVD_SDS_REPORT_2015.1_eng.pdf?ua=1&ua=1.

18. Morenike Folayan, Brandon Brown, Aminu Yakubu, Kristin Peterson, and Bridget Haire, "Compassionate use of experimental drugs in the Ebola outbreak," *Lancet* 384, no. 9957 (November 2014): 1843–44.

19. Michael Hay, David W. Thomas, John L. Craighead, Celia Economides, and Jesse Rosenthal, "Clinical development success rates for investigational drugs," *Nature Biotechnology* 32 (2014): 40–51.

20. What counts as a fair level of benefit for communities hosting research, and whether certain kinds of benefit must be provided (e.g., access to any proven effective interventions), is contested. See, for example, Participants in the 2001 Conference on Ethical Aspects of Research in Developing Countries, "Moral Standards for Research in Developing Countries: From 'Reasonable Availability' to 'Fair Benefits,'" *Hastings Center Report* 34 (2004): 17–27.

21. World Health Organization, "Ethical Considerations for Use of Unregistered Interventions for Ebola Viral Disease."

22. World Health Organization, "Ebola Response Roadmap," August 2014, accessed 7 July, 2015, http://www.who.int/csr/resources/publications/ebola/response-roadmap/en/.

23. Some commentators have noted the need to set priorities between the use of experimental interventions and containment and care, but the issue requires further discussion. See, for example, Annette Rid and Ezekiel J. Emanuel, "Ethical Considerations of Experimental Interventions in the Ebola Outbreak," *Lancet* 384, no. 9957 (November 2014): 1896–99; Arthur L. Arthur L. Caplan, "Morality in a Time of Ebola," *Lancet* 385, no. 9971 (March 2015): e16–e17; Angus J. Dawson, "Ebola: What It Tells Us about Medical Ethics," *Journal of Medical Ethics* 41, no.1 (January 2015): 107–10.

24. In addition, some argued that it was not only ethically acceptable to use the existing investigational vaccines or treatments, but obligatory to do so. For reasons of space, it is not possible to explore the surrounding questions here. See, for example, Caplan, "Morality in a Time of Ebola"; Bruce D. White, Luke C. Gelinas, and Wayne N. Shelton, "In Particular Circumstances Attempting Unproven Interventions is Permissible and Even Obligatory," *The American Journal of Bioethics* 15. No. 4 (2015): 53–55; Joshua T. Landry, Thomas Foreman, and Michael Kekewich, "Reconsidering the Ethical Permissibility of the Use of Unregistered Interventions against Ebola Virus Disease," *Cambridge Quarterly of Healthcare Ethics* 24, no. 3 (July 2015): 366–69.

25. World Health Organization, "Ethical considerations for use of unregistered interventions for Ebola viral disease." Readers should note, however, that a subsequent WHO Ethics Working Group concluded that experimental treatments "must be tested ... using ... simple but properly designed clinical trials." World Health Organization, "Ethical Issues Related to Study Design for Trials on Therapeutics for Ebola Virus Disease," WHO Ethics Working Group Meeting, October 21, 2014, accessed 7 July, 2015, http://www.who.int/medicines/wg_ethics_ebola_interventions/en/.

26. Steven Joffe, "Evaluating Novel Therapies during the Ebola Epidemic," *Journal of the American Medical Association* 312, no.13 (October 2014): 1299–1300; Annette Rid and Ezekiel J. Emanuel, "Compassionate Use of Experimental Drugs in the Ebola Outbreak—Authors' reply," *Lancet* 384, no. 9957 (November 2014): 1844; Andrew Hantel and Christoper Olusola Olopade, "Drug and Vaccine Access in the Ebola Epidemic: Advising Caution in Compassionate Use," *Annals of Internal Medicine* 162, no. 2 (January 2015): 141–42.

27. Seema K. Shah, David Wendler, and Marion Danis, "Examining the Ethics of Clinical Use of Unproven Interventions Outside of Clinical Trials during the Ebola Epidemic," *American Journal of Bioethics* 15, no. 4 (2015): 11–16.

28. This assumes that a relatively low number of interventions is deployed in experimental clinical care or prevention. If a large number were used, taking all interventions might not be feasible or may reduce their possible potential benefits due to interactive effects, in which case clinical trials would seem warranted.

29. Ezekiel J. Emanuel, David Wendler, and Christine Grady, "What Makes Clinical Research Ethical?" *Journal of the American Medical Association* 283, no. 20 (May 2000): 2701–11; Ezekiel J. Emanuel, David Wendler, Jack Killen, and Christine Grady, "What Makes Clinical Research in Developing Countries Ethical? The Benchmarks of Ethical Research," *Journal of Infectious Diseases* 189, no. 5 (2004): 930–37.

30. Rid and Emanuel, "Ethical considerations of experimental interventions in the Ebola outbreak."

31. For contributions on these issues in addition to the ones already cited in this paper, see, for example, Lawrence O. Gostin, "Ethical Allocation of Drugs and Vaccines in the West African Ebola Epidemic," *Milbank Quarterly* 92, no. 4 (December 2014): 662–66; Presidential Commission for the Study of Bioethical Issues, "Ethics and Ebola: Public Health Planning and Response," Washington, DC, February 2015, accessed 7 July 2015, http://bioethics.gov/node/4637; Jerome Amir Singh, "Humanitarian Access to Unapproved Interventions in Public Health Emergencies of International Concern," *PLoS Medicine* 12, no. 2 (February 2015): e1001793; Marc Lipsitch, Nir Eyal, M. Elizabeth Halloran, Miguel A. Hernán, Ira M. Longini, Eli N. Perencevich, et al., "Vaccine Testing: Ebola and Beyond," *Science* 348, no. 6230 (April 2015): 46–48; Robert Klitzman, "Evolving Challenges and Research Needs concerning Ebola," *American Journal of Public Health* (June 2015): e1-e3; Morenike Oluwatoyin Folayan, Brandon Brown, Bridget Haire, Aminu Yakubu, Kristin Peterson, and Jemee Tegli, "Stakeholders' Engagement with Ebola Therapy Research in Resource-Limited Settings," *BMC Infectious Diseases* 15, no. 1 (June 2015): 242.

32. Some representative contributions: Alex John London, "Clinical Research in a Public Health Crisis: The Integrative Approach Managing Uncertainty and Mitigating Conflict," *Seton Hall Law Review* 39, no. 4 (2009): 1173–1202; Ruth Macklin and Ethan Cowan, "Conducting Research in Disease Outbreaks," *PLOS Neglected Tropical Diseases* 3, no. 4 (2009): e335; Doris Schopper, Ross Upshur, Francine Matthys, Jerome Amir Singh, Sunita Sheel Bandewar, Aasim Ahmad, et al., "Research Ethics Review in Humanitarian Contexts: The Experience of the Independent Ethics Review Board of Médecins Sans Frontières," *PLOS Medicine* 6, no.7 (2009): e1000115; Nathan Ford, Edward J. Mills, Rony Zachariah, and Ross Upshur, "Ethics of Conducting Research in Conflict Settings," *Conflict and Health* 3, no.1 (2009): 7; Philippe Calain, Nathalie Fiore, Marc Poncin, and Samia Hurst, "Research Ethics and International Epidemic Response: The Case of Ebola and Marburg Hemorrhagic Fevers," *Public Health Ethics* 2, no.1 (2009): 7–29; Athula Sumathipala, Aamir Jafarey, Leonardo D. De Castro, Aasim Shmad, Darryl Marcer, Sandya

Srinivasan, et al., "Ethical Issues in Post-Disaster Clinical Interventions and Research: A Developing World Perspective; Key Findings from a Drafting and Consensus Generation Meeting of the Working Group on Disaster Research and Ethics," *Asian Bioethics Review* 2, no.2 (2010): 124–42; Dónal P. O'Mathúna, "Conducting Research in the Aftermath of Disasters: Ethical Considerations," *Journal of Evidence-Based Medicine* 3, no. 2 (2010): 65–75; Sarah J. L. Edwards, "Ethics of Clinical Science in a Public Health Emergency: Drug Discovery at the Bedside," *American Journal of Bioethics* 13, no. 9 (2013): 3–14; A. M. Viens, *Emergency Research Ethics* (Ashgate: Rumford, 2013).

33. Jesse L. Goodman "Studying 'Secret Serums'—Toward Safe, Effective Ebola Treatments," *The New England Journal of Medicine* 371, no. 12 (September 2014): 1086–89; Rid and Emanuel, "Ethical considerations of experimental interventions in the Ebola outbreak"; Joffe, "Evaluating novel therapies during the Ebola epidemic"; Edward Cox, Luciana Borio, and Robert Temple, "Evaluating Ebola Therapies—The Case for RCTs," *The New England Journal of Medicine* 371, no. 25 (December 2014): 2350–51.

34. Clement Adebamowo, Oumou Bah-Sow, Fred Binka, Roberto Bruzzone, Arthur Caplan, Jean-François Delfraissy, et al., "Randomised Controlled Trials for Ebola: Practical and Ethical Issues," *Lancet* 384, no. 9952 (October 2014): 1423–24; Arthur L. Caplan, Carolyn Plunkett, and Bruce Levin, "Selecting the Right Tool for the Job," *The American Journal of Bioethics* 15, no.4 (2015): 4–10. A good overview of the controversy is offered by Jon Cohen, "Issues Continue to Dog the Testing of Ebola Drugs and Vaccines," *Science Magazine*, 16 October 2014, http://news.sciencemag.org/health/2014/10/issues-continue-dog-testing-ebola-drugs-and-vaccines.

35. World Health Organization, "Ethical issues related to study design for trials on therapeutics for Ebola Virus Disease."

36. Emanuel et al., "What Makes Clinical Research Ethical?"; Emanuel et al., "What Makes Clinical Research in Developing Countries Ethical?"

37. Emanuel et al., "What Makes Clinical Research Ethical?"; Emanuel et al., "What Makes Clinical Research in Developing Countries Ethical?"; Rid and Wendler, "A Framework for Risk-Benefit Evaluations in Biomedical Research."

38. Adebamowo et al., "Randomised Controlled Trials for Ebola"; Caplan et al., "Selecting the Right Tool for the Job."

39. Rashid Ansumana, Kathryn H. Jacobsen, M'baimba Idris, Henry Bangura, Mohamed Boie-Jalloh, Joseph M. Lamin, et al., "Ebola in Freetown Area, Sierra Leone—A Case Study of 581 Patients," *New England Journal of Medicine* 372, no.6 (December 2014): 587–88. For a more extensive review of the available data on mortality rates in the 2014 Ebola outbreak, see Annette Rid, "The Goals of Research during an Epidemic," *The American Journal of Bioethics* 15, no. 4 (2015): 47–50.

40. Donald G. McNeil, "Ebola Doctors Are Divided on IV Therapy in Africa," *The New York Times*, January 1, 2015, http://www.nytimes.com/2015/01/02/health/ebola-doctors-are-divided-on-iv-therapy-in-africa.html.

41. Emanuel et al., "What Makes Clinical Research Ethical?"; Emanuel et al., "What Makes Clinical Research in Developing Countries Ethical?"; Annette Rid and David Wendler, "A Framework for Risk-Benefit Evaluations in Biomedical Research," *Kennedy Institute of Ethics Journal* 21, no. 2 (June 2011): 141–79.

42. Steven Joffe and Franklin G. Miller, "Bench to Bedside: Mapping the Moral Terrain of Clinical Research," *Hastings Center Report* 38, no. 2 (2008): 30–42; Rid and Wendler, "A Framework for Risk-Benefit Evaluations in Biomedical Research."

43. Emanuel et al., "What Makes Clinical Research Ethical?"; Emanuel et al., "What Makes Clinical Research in Developing Countries Ethical?"

44. Joffe, "Evaluating Novel Therapies during the Ebola Epidemic."

15 History, Culture, and Social Norms: Implications for Ebola Drug and Vaccine Clinical Trials

Morenike Oluwatoyin Folayan and Bridget Haire

The quantity of literature published during the months that followed the Ebola virus disease (EVD) outbreak in West Africa was unprecedented in the history of a disease identified almost 40 years ago. The magnitude of the outbreak in West Africa, which started in December 2013 and was on the decline as of July 2015,[1] makes it clear that while countries in the "Ebola zone" have borne the brunt of the epidemic, the impact of the outbreak is global.

The EVD epidemic precipitated debates about the appropriate methodologies for conducting clinical trials of drugs and vaccines during a major infectious disease outbreak. Urgency regarding drug development was intensified by news reports demonstrating the appalling conditions in which people with EVD are treated and health care workers are expected to work. Controversies about drug development processes were exacerbated by news that ZMapp, an investigational agent available in very limited supply, was accessible to foreign nationals but inaccessible to Africans worst affected by the disease.[2]

While the research for EVD treatments and vaccines is urgent, research priorities cannot be allowed to divert resources from critical patient care and public health activities, as proven interventions should be funded ahead of research in order to resolve the crisis.[3] This makes the process by which research is incorporated into the battle for survival of patients with EVD of the greatest practical and moral importance. The paucity of health care delivery systems in most parts of Africa renders decision making about EVD drug and vaccine trial designs hugely significant. First, there is the need to know whether experimental therapies increase survival. Second, there is the "rule of rescue,"[4] which supports the use of any plausible and available treatment to reduce mortality and morbidity. This is applicable in the context of EVD management given the extreme suffering experienced by people infected with EVD. Finally, it is necessary to evaluate what therapies or vaccines work best among the experimental candidates. Together, these considerations mean that there are complex decisions to be made about the design and implementation of EVD clinical research.

We will argue in this chapter for the necessity to be open to a range of methodological approaches to EVD clinical research and to ensure community-consultation mechanisms are in place to help shape the design and implementation of EVD-related clinical research. We also argue for the need to ensure post-trial benefits for affected communities and the need to strengthen the health care systems through investments made during the EVD research process.

EVD and the Controversy over Randomized Controlled Trials

Broadly perceived to produce objective, unbiased evidence of the highest quality, randomized controlled trials (RCTs) are frequently described as the "gold standard" of research. This belief is particularly strong for double-blinded RCTs, where neither the participants nor the researcher knows whether the randomization is to an active drug or a placebo/standard of care. It has been argued that RCTs are the best way to maximize social values and the scientific validity of EVD clinical research,[5] and that the benefits of randomization are so substantial every opportunity to use RCTs should be taken.[6] For regulatory purposes, RCTs are required to provide the needed evidence to draw conclusions about drug safety and efficacy for licensing.[7]

The RCT methodology, however, has been criticized for requiring that the best interests of current patients be sacrificed, via random allocation to different study arms, for the best interests of future patients who will benefit from the knowledge produced by the study.[8] Many therefore consider that RCTs are justified only in conditions of clinical equipoise: where the relevant scientific or medical community holds, on reasonable grounds, that the superiority of an experimental agent has not been established.[9] Equipoise is broadly acknowledged as the moral justification for randomization in health care research, as the interests of participants are not "sacrificed" in the case where the difference between treatment modalities is unknown.[10]

Dawson[11] argues that EVD clinical trials present a situation of genuine uncertainty, and therefore justify randomization to experimental treatment versus control. However, we argue that while there may be equipoise for EVD clinical trials, equipoise may not be a sufficient moral justification for randomization for EVD clinical trials in the absence of an effective standard of care for EVD;[12] in the presence of high patient mortality;[13] and when there are alternate experimental options that provide useful data.[14]

Unfortunately, much of the dialogue about clinical trial design for EVD drug and vaccine research has been driven by biomedical perspectives of appropriate clinical trial designs and how best to determine the efficacy and effectiveness of the experimental products. Little consideration has been given to the historical, political, and social context of the lives of those worst affected by EVD, which could impact the recruitment, retention, and use of EVD therapies and are factors that would affect the success of any clinical trial conducted, irrespective of design. This is significant, because EVD is a disease of poverty and neglected health systems.[15] The current global emphasis has, unfortunately, not focused on addressing the drivers of EVD, thereby potentiating future outbreaks in a socioeconomic context that places affected nations at risk of not being able to purchase the developed EVD drugs or vaccines without donor support.

This chapter takes a look at the historical, cultural, and social context of the lives of the population worst affected by EVD and the implications for the design and implementation of EVD drug clinical trials. However, we recognize that for effective responses for EVD management and control in the affected region, a lot more needs to be done than investing in EVD drug and vaccine development: Many of these structural factors, which are of public health importance, would also affect access to and uptake of EVD treatment and vaccines when developed.

History, the State, and Implications for EVD Response

Sierra Leone and Liberia have both been affected by many years of civil war, and Guinea has suffered many years of coups and political violence. The civil disruption in these countries left political systems fragile with citizens who are sensitive to signals of marginalization. Journalists report antagonism toward the political system in these countries, resulting from the unresponsiveness of political elites to the needs of citizens and the failure to care enough for society.[16] The relationship of citizens with government is plagued with distrust and feelings of abandonment and frustration. Against this backdrop, the EVD epidemic underscored the existing social and political tensions and undermined the cooperation required for effective public health responses. Health workers on strike from an Ebola treatment unit, who were promised but then denied increased pay for risking their lives, is but one example of this tension.[17]

There is also a history of distrust of foreign nationals promulgated by the government following the incursion of foreigners into domestic politics in the wake of humanitarian and refugee programs that followed the period of civil crisis.[18] This distrust of "foreign elements" is exemplified by local attacks on a Médecins Sans Frontières treatment center in Guinea, and denial of access to foreign NGOs and government agents in some settlements during the epidemic.[19] This distrust is a potential source of crisis during EVD research if the research is perceived as exploitative or perpetuating inequity.[20]

Civil disruptions have had negative impacts on health and health care costs well beyond the conflict period.[21] Conflict typically disrupts economic activity, reduces access to clean water and food, and diverts resources from health care.[22] It also results in breakdown of systems for public health surveillance, epidemic outbreak monitoring, and health communication networks,[23] with associated increases in incidence of infectious disease[24] and disease-related deaths.[25] Conflict also results in the loss of health professionals to death, injury, or emigration; disruption of governance structures and supply lines; and interruption of health campaigns, in addition to increased demands for care.[26] This is exemplified by the low ranking of Sierra Leone, Liberia, and Guinea on the human development index.[27] These weakened health care systems became nonresponsive during the Ebola epidemic. The gaps were so egregious that the system itself became a vector for the spread of the disease.[28]

Post-wartime, countries in the Ebola zone experienced recurrent outbreaks of infectious diseases such as cholera, yellow fever, Lassa fever, dengue fever, typhoid,[29] measles, and meningitis.[30] The control of these infectious disease outbreaks has always depended on response and support from the international community. However, at the time of the EVD outbreak, "donor fatigue" had set in, and the international community was engaged in setting up fledgling systems to reduce donor dependency.[31] The fragile transitional systems were unable to handle the EVD outbreak, because it was outside routine health care management.[32] The lateness of the response from the international community, combined with the decentralization of a health care system that could have helped facilitate an EVD surveillance response, further contributed to poor epidemic control. Indigenous responses also required that changes be made to routine state activities, with implications for political, social and economic changes.[33] These changes take time and resulted in further delays in state response to the epidemic.

Culture, Social Norms, and the Implications for EVD Research

Local values—including culture and social norms—are an essential factor in making a decision about the selection of drugs that move though clinical testing.[34] There is, however, very little debate about how local values can influence EVD drug trial design. Waldman and Nieburg[35] rightly acknowledge that with EVD crisis management, *Western scientific thinking has been forced to confront the realities of other cultures*. Where attitudes toward prevention of illness and their treatment collide, as is expected in situations with EVD management, proposals that make significant efforts to incorporate scientific and local values have the best chance for success.

As an example of how culture and international scientific research are necessarily intertwined, Zvonareva et al.[36] provide empirical data to show how South African participants in international research viewed their participation as a contribution toward the collective benefit of the community. To the participants, research was a form of partnership between communities and researchers with the aim of achieving better health. Sociocultural practices and understandings validate or invalidate the practice of science and how community members make sense of the clinical trial process.[37] Local community perspectives of research are also informed by indigenous accounts of what is right and wrong.[38] A history of colonial exploitation, foreigners driving the EVD research process, and the prospect of benefits derivable from a clinical trial process have significant import for shaping connotations, perspectives, and reporting of the EVD epidemic in the local histories of these communities.

While there are biomedical perspectives about the science and ethics of clinical trial design, values rooted in culture and local moral traditions influence research participation.[39] For this reason, it is an ethical imperative to have visible, meaningful local input in the design of the response to the EVD epidemic to ensure the research is understood as ethical and humanely focused and does not violate harmonious relationships within the society. When there are differences in ethical perspective between cultures, parties must engage and negotiate to resolve these differences.[40] The importance of collaborative research that remains cognizant of social values and respects legitimate ethical expectations of research participants can therefore not be overemphasized.

Design and Implementation of EVD Clinical Trials in EVD-Affected Countries

For the most part, EVD drug and vaccine clinical trials would be classified as international research conducted in resource-limited settings. Concerns therefore arise about beneficiaries of the outcome of research: Researchers advance their careers, pharmaceutical companies make gains, and citizens in the resource-poor Ebola zone would have to contend with the World Trade Organization Agreement on Trade-Related Aspects of Intellectual Property Rights to access EVD drugs and vaccines when developed. How then can people affected by EVD benefit from EVD research in the short, medium, and long term?

There are four possible ways that this could be achieved, namely: (1) ensure study protocols are developed in consultation with local researchers; (2) prioritize community engagement throughout the research design and implementation process; (3) establish concrete plans regarding future access to EVD drugs during future outbreaks; and (4) foster investment in health care infrastructure. We consider these processes to be mechanisms through which EVD research can be sensitive to the histories, cultures, and social norms of the respective communities, thereby promoting co-ownership of the EVD research process.

Study Protocols

EVD study protocols should be developed in collaboration with researchers who work in countries where studies are to be conducted. Local researchers should be intellectually invested in the planning and implementation of the research from its conceptualizing through to its implementation, data analysis, and data interpretation.

Engagement of local researchers in the design of EVD research allows for in-country discussions on study specimen ownership, study specimen shipment process, and data sharing prior to biobanking. This process also helps ensure that local social, political, and cultural perspectives inform the design of clinical trials. Acknowledging the legitimacy of cultural norms should promote exploration of alternative research designs that can produce desired outcomes with levels of scientific validity similar to what would be expected for more traditional clinical trial designs.

Possible alternative research designs proposed for testing Ebola interventions include a cluster-randomized trial, wherein different therapies are offered in parallel at different sites.[41] This design requires (a) that a consistent standard of care is applied rigorously at each trial site, and (b) the experimental therapies have a significant enough impact that the "noise" in the statistical analysis is outweighed by a dramatic reduction in mortality. Unfortunately, the first condition is very challenging to achieve with the current EVD epidemic in West Africa, and the second condition is unlikely to be met.

A second possibility is the sequential randomized control trial (SRCT) design,[42] wherein randomization occurs at the group (health service) level, with active experimental treatments available to all participants. The trial has built-in adaptation features, so that if or when a treatment shows superior results, more participants could be switched to that intervention. Data would be collected using an observational protocol. Again, this design requires consistent and agreed-upon standards of nonexperimental care between sites, with failure to achieve this being a confounder.

A third possibility is the use of a multistage approach (MSA) including both nonrandomized and randomized elements. When the outcomes of the MSA approach were compared to SRCT and conventional RCT, both the MSA and SRCT led to substantially fewer deaths than a conventional RCT if the tested interventions were either highly effective or harmful.[43] One major threat to the validity of the results of the non-randomized components of the MSA, as mentioned, is the inability to ensure the consistency of the standard of care provided to patients at the treatment sites.

A further alternative EVD vaccine trial design is the "stepped-wedge" trial design, in which randomization occurs at the group or community level, and each group eventually receives the intervention in a staggered, step-wise timeline.[44] Similar adaptive non-randomized clinical trial designs are being implemented for ongoing EVD vaccines clinical trials.

An example of stepped-wedge trial design is the alternative "ring" design used in Guinea to determine the efficacy of a recombinant, replication-competent vesicular stomatitis virus-based vaccine in the phase III *Ebola ça Suffit* trial.[45] The study actively recruited every person who had come into contact with an Ebola-infected person for vaccination with the experimental product: Some were offered vaccination immediately, while others received the vaccination after 21 days delay. The interim results showed that the study product was 100% protective in the group that was immediately vaccinated. While true vaccine efficacy is likely to be lower than that figure, as vaccines that produce sterilizing immunity are extremely rare, the study result suggest the tested candidate vaccine is likely to be effective at the population level. The outcome of the *Ebola ça Suffit* trial justifies the use of alternative clinical trial designs to establish the efficacy of a candidate product during a critical emergency health crisis.

Community Engagement

The community engagement process should promote public dialogue to address misconceptions; foster equity and justice in participant selection, recruitment, and retention strategies; and encourage honest discussions about risks, benefits, and future drug and vaccine access.[46] It should also help community advocates become knowledgeable about scientific aspects of proposed trials in order to contribute meaningfully to discussions about clinical trial design.[47] Public dialogue facilitates the design of culturally sensitive and politically appropriate clinical-trial implementation processes. Such public dialogue should engage researchers and community representatives affected by current and past EVD epidemics, since their experiences help enrich the research design process. Community partnership with researchers would have significant impact on the future narrative of the EVD response in local community histories.[48] Dialogue helps shape perception of clinical research.[49]

Future Drug Access

Concrete plans need to be made to ensure access to EVD drugs during future EVD outbreaks. This would help to avoid exploitation of countries and citizens that have invested human resources in the EVD drugs trials. The Declaration of Helsinki and the Council for International Organizations of Medical Sciences ethical guidelines stipulate that research protocols submitted to ethics committee for review must discuss post-trial access to experimental products. The determination of the efficacy or effectiveness of EVD drugs and vaccines cannot be the end of EVD researchers' investment in the EVD response. EVD clinical trials need to be planned with the view of ensuring future access to developed drugs for regions that participated in the research. We recognize that planning for post-trial access to an as-yet unlicensed product is difficult: There may be no plan for manufacture or scale-up. This highlights the need for public-private partnerships to ensure production in the event that a product is shown safe and effective. In this, pharmaceutical firms ought to be credited with proactively engaging in the development of EVD vaccines[50] and drug development in collaboration with government agencies and academic institutions.

Health Care Infrastructure

While we do appreciate that it is the state's responsibility to address health care provision for its citizens, we feel that research enterprises that conduct clinical trials in countries affected by EVD epidemics have a moral duty to invest in building health care systems and structures. Such efforts would contribute to long-term human and infrastructural development for future research in neglected tropical diseases. The current EVD epidemic shows the global community that these neglected diseases have the potential to escalate to become global health security threats[51] when health systems fail. Investing in developing effective health systems in the region prior to the next crisis should be a priority of the global collective.[52] This would enhance EVD treatment and vaccine research that needs to take place during the next EVD outbreak.[53] The global commitment to health security and health research should inevitably lead to the commitment of research projects to strengthen the health systems within which EVD clinical trials are conducted.

There are propositions that the limited available resources for EVD management and control should be invested in strengthening the health care system rather than EVD research.[54] While we do not believe in an "either/or" approach for EVD management and control, we do strongly agree on the need to mobilize local resources and empower local people to provide the required care needed to increase the chances of survival of EVD patients vis à vis prompt diagnosis; intensive supportive treatment within a health care facility; and critical public health interventions, such as contact tracing, isolation, surveillance, safe burial, and effective community engagement.

Conclusion

The design and implementation of research that establishes the efficacy and effectiveness of EVD drugs and vaccines is important. RCTs are widely recognized to address these questions, but may not always be appropriate for use in a crisis situation when there is an urgent need to treat large numbers of people[55] and to establish ways for people to better protect themselves from infection. It is possible to generate evidence about the effectiveness of EVD drug therapy and vaccines without the ethical and moral challenges associated with standard RCT design.

The options for drug and vaccine clinical trials should not only be informed by science, but also by the history, politics, culture, and social norms of the communities to be engaged in clinical trials. Trial design for EVD research should promote equity in experimental drug access during an epidemic with high case fatality, especially in the face of a history of inequitable access to experimental interventions (e.g., ZMapp), past colonial exploitation, distrust of foreigners, differing local understandings of ethics, and the collegial expectations of sharing outcomes of research.

EVD drug and vaccine researchers should explore the suitability of alternative approaches to RCTs for conducting clinical trials in EVD-affected zones. Study designs must also include best supportive care, even if it is not locally available. The known standard of care for EVD management should not be denied patients enrolled in clinical trials, regardless of the local context of where the study is conducted. Finally, our argument for alternative clinical trial designs does not the preclude the implementation of conventional RCTs for the investigation of EVD drugs and vaccines during an EVD epidemic where supportive therapy is optimal, health systems are efficient, research literacy is high, community understanding and perception of biomedical ethics align perfectly with researchers' perspectives, and there is no history of exploitation and distrust of foreigners.

Acknowledgments

The dialogues on the ethics of Ebola management we held with our colleagues, with whom we worked between 2014 and 2015, shaped our thoughts for this manuscript: Aminu Yakubu, Brandon Brown, Jamee Tegli, and Kristin Peterson. We also thank Liza Dawson and Patricia Kingori for finding time to critically review the manuscript and providing useful comments.

Notes

1. World Health Organization, "Ebola Situation Report—27 May 2015," http://www.who.int/csr/disease/ebola/situation-reports/archive/en.

2. Adia Benton, "Race and the Immuno-logics of Ebola Response in West Africa," Somatosphere (blog), September 19, 2014, http://somatosphere.net/2014/09/race-and-the-immuno-logics-of-ebola-response-in-west-africa.html.

3. Arthur L. Caplan, "Morality in a Time of Ebola," *Lancet* 385, no. 9971 (2015): e16-e17.

4. Albert Jonsen, "Bentham in a Box: Technology Assessment and Health Care Allocation," *Law, Medicine and Health Care* 14, no. 3–4 (1986): 172–75.

5. Annette Rid and E. J. Emanuel, "Ethical Considerations of Experimental Interventions in The Ebola Outbreak," *Lancet* 384, no. 9957 (2014): 1896–9; Steven Joffe, "Evaluating Novel Therapies during the Ebola Epidemic," *Journal of the American Medical Association* 312, no. 13 (2014): 1299–1300.

6. Thomas A. Louis, "Expand the Toolkit!" *American Journal of Bioethics* 15, no. 4 (2015): 40–42.

7. Robert M. Nelson, Michelle Roth-Clinea, Kevin Prohaskaa, Edward Coxa, Luciana Borioa, and Robert Templea, "Right Job, Wrong Tool: A Commentary on Designing Clinical Trials for EVD," *American Journal of Bioethics* 15, no. 4 (2015): 33–36.

8. Sarah Edwards, David A. Braunholtz, Richard J. Lilford, and Andrew J. Stevens, "Ethical Issues in the Design and Conduct of Cluster Randomized Controlled Trials," *BMJ* 22, no. 318 (1999): 1407–9.

9. Benjamin Freedman, "Equipoise and the Ethics of Clinical Research," *New England Journal of Medicine* 317, no. 3 (1987): 141–4.

10. Though not universally; see e.g., Franklin G. Miller and H. Brody, "A Critique of Clinical Equipoise: Therapeutic Misconception in the Ethics of Clinical Trials,"*Hastings Center Report* 33, no. 3 (2003): 19–28; Franklin G. Miller and H.

Brody, "Clinical Equipoise and the Incoherence of Research Ethics," *Journal of Medicine and Philosophy* 32, no. 2 (2007):151–65.

11. Liza Dawson, "Not all RCTs Are Created Equal: Lessons from Early AIDS Trials," *American Journal of Bioethics* 15, no. 4 (2015): 45–47.

12. Donald G. McNeil, "Ebola Doctors Are Divided on IV Therapy in Africa," *TheNew York Times*, January 1, 2015, http://www.nytimes.com/2015/01/02/health/ebola-doctors-are-divided-on-iv-therapy-in-africa.html.

13. Chris Degeling, J. Johnson, and C. Mayes, "Impure Politics and Pure Science: Efficacious Ebola Medications Are Only a Palliation and Not a Cure for Structural Disadvantage," *American Journal of Bioethics* 15, no. 4 (2015): 43–45.

14. Arthur L. Caplan, C. Plunkett, and B. Levin, "Selecting the Right Tool for the Job," *American Journal of Bioethics* 15, no. 4 (2015): 4–10.

15. Peter Piot, *No Time to Lose: A Life in Pursuit of Deadly Viruses* (New York: W. W. Norton, 2012).

16. Johanna Söderström, "Ebola and the Ex-Combatant Community," Cultural Anthropology Online, October 07, 2014, http://www.culanth.org/fieldsights/601-ebola-and-the-ex-combatant-community.

17. *The Telegraph*, "Liberia Health Workers Strike over Ebola 'Danger Money,'" October 13, 2014, http://www.telegraph.co.uk/news/worldnews/ebola/11159217/Liberia-health-workers-strike-over-Ebola-danger-money.html.

18. Anita Schroven, "Ebola in Guinea: Revealing the State of the State," Cultural Anthropology Online, October 07, 2014, http://www.culanth.org/fieldsights/587-ebola-in-guinea-revealing-the-state-of-the-state.

19. Ibid.

20. Johanna Söderström, "Ebola and the Ex-Combatant Community."

21. Ramon Sabes-Figuera, Paul McCrone, Marija Bogic, Dean Ajdukovic, Tanja Franciskovic, and Niccolò Colombini, et al., "Long-Term Impact of War on Health Care Costs: An Eight-Country Study," *PLoS One* 7, no. 1 (2012): e29603; Hazem A. Ghobarah, B.P. Huth, and C.B. Russett, "The Post-War Public Health Effects of Civil Conflict," *Social Science and Medicine* 59 (2004): 869–84.

22. Hazem A. Ghobarah, B.P. Huth, and C.B. Russett, "The Post-War Public Health Effects of Civil Conflict," *Social Science and Medicine* 59 (2004): 869–84.

23. Sharon A. Abramowitz, "How the Liberian Health Sector Became a Vector for Ebola," Cultural Anthropology Online, October 7, 2014, http://www.culanth.org/fieldsights/598-how-theliberian-health-sector-became-a-vector-for-ebola.

24. Michael J. Toole, "Complex Emergencies: Refugee and Other Populations," in *The Public Health Consequences of Disasters*, ed. E. Noji (New York: Oxford University Press, 1997).

25. P. Gustafson, Victor Francisco Gomes, C. S. Vieira, and Peter Aaby, "Tuberculosis Mortality during a Civil War in Guinea-Bissau," *Journal of the American Medical Association* 286 (2001): 599–603; David Heymann, Lincoln Chen, Keizo Takemi, David P. Fidler, Jordan W. Tappero, Mathew J. Thomas, et al., "Global Health Security: The Wider Lessons from the West African Ebola Virus Disease Epidemic," *Lancet* 385 (2015): 1894–6.

26. Heymann, et al., "Global Health Security: The Wider Lessons from the West African Ebola Virus Disease Epidemic."

27. United Nations Development Programme, "Human Development Report—The Rise of the South: Human Progress in a Diverse World," 2013, http://www.undp.org/content/undp/en/home/librarypage/hdr/human-development-report-2013.html.

28. Abramowitz, "How the Liberian Health Sector Became a Vector for Ebola."

29. Ibid.

30. Schroven, "Ebola in Guinea: Revealing the State of the State."

31. Abramowitz, "How the Liberian Health Sector Became a Vector for Ebola."

32. Schroven, "Ebola in Guinea: Revealing the State of the State."

33. Ibid.

34. Arthur L. Caplan, C. Plunkett, and B. Levin, "The Perfect Must Not Overwhelm the Good: Response to Open Peer Commentaries on 'Selecting the Right Tool For the Job,'" *The American Journal of Bioethics* 15, no. 4 (2015): W8–W10.

35. Waldman and Nieburg, "Thoughts on Alternative Designs for Clinical Trials for Ebola Treatment Research," 38–40.

36. Olga Zvonareva, Nora Engel, Eleanor Ross, Ron Berghmans, Ames Dhai, andAnja Krumeich, "Engaging Diverse Social and Cultural Worlds: Perspectives on Benefits in International Clinical Research from South African Communities," *Developing World Bioethics* 15 (2015): 8–17.

37. Sheila Jasanoff, "Technologies and Humility," *Nature* 450 (2007): 33.

38. Zvonareva et al., "Engaging Diverse Social and Cultural Worlds: Perspectives on Benefits in International Clinical Research from South African Communities."

39. Nicholas A. Christakis, "Ethics Are Local: Engaging Cross-Cultural Variation in the Ethics for Clinical Research," *Social Science and Medicine* 35 (1992): 1079–91.

40. Ibid.

41. Clement Adebamowo, Oumou Bah-Sow, Fred Binka, Roberto Bruzzone, Arthur Caplan, Jean-François Delfraissy, et al., "Randomised Controlled Trials for Ebola: Practical and Ethical Issues," *Lancet* 384, no. 9952 (2014):1423–4, doi: 10.1016/S0140-6736(14)61734-7.

42. Caplan, Plunkett, and Levin, "Selecting the Right Tool for the Job," 4–10.

43. Ben S. Cooper, Maciej F. Boni, Wirichada Pan-ngum, Nicholas P. J. Day, Peter W. Horby, Piero Olliaro, et al., "Evaluating Clinical Trial Designs for Investigational Treatments of Ebola Virus Disease," *PLoS Medicine* 12 (2015): e1001815.

44. Kanapathipillai Rupa, Ana Maria Henao Restrepo, Patricia Fast, David Wood, Christopher Dye, Marie-Paule Kieny, et al., "Ebola Vaccine: An Urgent International Priority," *New England Journal of Medicine* 371 (2014): 2249–51.

45. Ana Maria Henao-Restrepo, Ira M. Longini, Matthias Egger,Natalie E. Dean, W. John Edmunds, Anton Camacho, et al., "Efficacy and Effectiveness of an rVSV-Vectored Vaccine Expressing Ebola Surface Glycoprotein: Interim Results from the Guinea Ring Vaccination Cluster-Randomized Trial," *Lancet* 386, no. 9996 (2015), 857–66.

46. Morenike Oluwatoyin Folayan, Brandon Brown, Bridget Haire, Aminu Yakubu, Kristin Peterson, and Jemee Tegli, "Stakeholders' Engagement with Ebola Therapy Research in Resource Limited Settings," *BMC Infectious Diseases* 15, no. 242 (2015). doi: 10.1186/s12879-015-0950-8.

47. Dawson, "Not all RCTs Are Created Equal: Lessons from Early AIDS Trials," 45–47.

48. Steven Epstein, *Impure Science: AIDS, Activism, and the Politics of Knowledge* (Berkeley: University of California Press, 1996).

49. Zvonareva et al., "Engaging Diverse Social and Cultural Worlds: Perspectives on Benefits in International Clinical Research from South African Communities."

50. Folayan, "Stakeholder Engagement and Ebola Virus Disease Therapy Research," 2015.

51. Ibid.

52. Ibid.

53. Miriam Shuchman, "Ebola Vaccine Trial in West Africa Faces Criticism," *Lancet* 385 (2015): 1933–4.

54. Francois Lamontagne, Christophe Clément, Thomas Fletcher, Shevin T. Jacob, William A. Fischer II, and Robert A. Fowler, "Doing Today's Work Superbly Well—Treating Ebola with Current Tools," *New England Journal of Medicine* 371, no. 17

(2014): 1565–6; Christopher J.M. Whitty, Jeremy Farrar, Neil Ferguson, W. John Edmunds, Peter Piot, Melissa Leach, et al., "Infectious Disease: Tough Choices to Reduce Ebola Transmission," *Nature* 515, no. 7526 (2014): 192–4; Joseph Millum, "Controlling Ebola Trials," *American Journal of Bioethics* 15, no. 4 (2015): 36–37.

55. Degeling, Johnson, and Mayes, "Impure Politics and Pure Science: Efficacious Ebola Medications Are Only a Palliation and Not a Cure for Structural Disadvantage," 43–45; Dawson, "Not all RCTs Are Created Equal: Lessons from Early AIDS Trials," 45–47.

16 Rejecting Quarantine: A Frozen-in-Time Reaction to Disease

Kelly Hills

On October 1, 2014, America awoke to an unwelcome surprise: A patient had been diagnosed with Ebola virus disease (EVD) in Texas. Surprise quickly turned to fear as people wondered what their risk was, and this risk turned to the question of quarantine. Who should be quarantined? Should everyone from Africa be quarantined? Everyone from EVD-affected countries? What constituted a case of EVD worth quarantining? Should everyone be quarantined, kept either in or out depending on your perspective? Should all medical workers be quarantined? And although all medical information stated that EVD is not contagious until symptoms manifest and quarantine is an overreaction, at no point did anyone stop to ask the simpler question: Should quarantine be a part of our disease response at all? The answer to this is no: Quarantine in the modern era is predominantly an outdated, unjustifiable violation of an individual's rights to justice, autonomy, privacy, and liberty. It is, I contend, no longer a viable response to infectious disease.

To begin, it is helpful to distinguish between isolation and quarantine. The two are quite separate in concept and should remain so in discussion: Quarantine is a coercive social-distancing model that removes those who have been exposed to disease and might become sick, but who have not tested positive for disease or manifested clinical symptoms of disease, from the community.[1] Isolation removes those who are confirmed sick from the population for treatment and recovery.[2] But is it really accurate to call isolation coercive social distancing when you're sick? As Annas notes, "as a general rule, sick people seek treatment."[3] Because of this voluntary seeking of medical assistance, anyone who is then admitted to an isolation ward is there because they have an interest in getting better.[4]

Likewise, most people do not want to infect those around them, especially family members, and will voluntarily seek out health care and follow reasonable public health advice to avoid spreading disease. The key here, of course, is what constitutes "reasonable public health," and whether or not the people determining the definitions agree with the people who are expected to live out these definitions.

Quarantine is an epidemic story[5]—but as the media frenzy in the United States showed, an epidemic is not necessary in order to have the epidemic story of quarantine. As such, and before discussing the history, use, and limits of quarantine, it will be helpful to have several stories.

Thomas Eric Duncan

On September 26, 2014, Thomas Eric Duncan went to a Dallas-area hospital with abdominal pain, dizziness, nausea, and headaches. When he was evaluated, his temperature was noted at 100°F; he was otherwise medically unremarkable. Although the hospital had implemented policy, over a month earlier, asking that all patients complete a travel history, the medical record indicates that the triage nurse did not obtain this information from Duncan, and thus missed the fact that he had recently arrived in America from Liberia. Duncan was diagnosed with "sinusitis and abdominal pain" and discharged. He continued to sicken and returned to the hospital on September 30, when he was properly diagnosed with EVD. He died October 8, 2014—the only person to have died of EVD in America to date.[6]

Duncan's fiancée Louise Troh, their son, and two nephews were forcibly quarantined in an apartment that contained soiled blankets and towels so likely to be contaminated with EVD that Texas could not find a company with appropriate permits to transport the biohazardous waste.[7] Despite caring for Duncan the entire time he was ill, and remaining in the contaminated apartment for several days before being moved, Troh, her son, and her nephews did not became sick.

Craig Spencer

Spencer returned to America on October 17, 2014, after working with Doctors Without Borders in Guinea. He entered the country through JFK International Airport in New York City and showed no symptoms of EVD. Spencer did not undergo voluntary quarantine while home in New York

City, but he did monitor his vital signs and symptoms twice a day. He began to feel sick and run a fever on Thursday, October 23, and reported to a hospital, where he was diagnosed with EVD.[8] Even though Spencer spent significant time with two friends and lived with his fiancée, all of whom were involuntarily quarantined at home, no one was infected by him.[9]

Kaci Hickox

On October 24, 2014, Kaci Hickox returned to American after a month working with EVD patients in Sierra Leone. She arrived at Newark International Airport, in New Jersey, on the same day that the governors of New York and New Jersey began mandatory quarantine of all medical workers returning from Western African nations.[10] Although she showed no signs of illness and there was no medical concern that she was ill, Hickox was quarantined in a tent with no heat, television, shower, or portable toilet.[11] She was originally told that she would be kept in this involuntary quarantine for 21 days. Instead, Hickox fought, was released, and traveled to Maine, where she continued self-surveillance and voluntary quarantine while fighting the quarantine efforts in courts.[12]

These stories give us some background to the lack of scientific fact behind the quarantine impulse, as well as highlight the outsized influence politicians and elections had on public health policy implementation.

A Brief History of Quarantine

In order to discuss the present use of quarantine, it is helpful to look to the past and our history with the term and action. In all likelihood, most people will be familiar with the public health narrative that places quarantine as an artifact of 1348 Venice, an action of Doge Andrea Dandolo and the Venetian Great Council[13] to stem the effects of the plague on the city of Venice. While it is likely that some form of removing from society those who have been exposed to illness existed before this, most historical accounts focus instead on separating those who are already ill: that is, what we contemporarily refer to as isolation. Leviticus 13 goes into great detail about both when to isolate a patient and, if the infected person survives, when they can be released back into the community. Lazarettos, hospitals for lepers—often beyond city limits—existed in Europe in the late seventh century, and served as both a place to contain lepers and a place for treatment. And in a time where illness was often seen as divine punishment for transgressions, it was not uncommon for those who were sick to be driven out of society.[14]

What was different about Venice was that the effort to prevent plague moved beyond isolation of the sick to isolation of those who posed a threat of illness to society: sailors. Those aboard merchant ships could have been exposed to plague before getting on the ship and not yet be manifesting the symptoms. In order to protect the city, the Doge and Great Council ordered all ships held offshore for a period of time[15] before entering the city proper. Other cities saw the virtue of Venice's actions and followed suit over the next century;[16] by 1374, the holding period was set at a biblically inspired forty days.[17] Inspired by port cities, inland cities set up *cordon sanitaires*, a controlled border around a town that expressively forbade travel to or from plague-stricken areas without special dispensation from city elders.[18]

Two related things should stand out to any reader when discussing the history of quarantine. First, quarantine was established at a time where the cutting-edge theory of contagion was miasma. According to this theory, disease originated in the environment and was caused by decaying organic matter that released a poisonous air or rotting vapor, causing infection in weak or susceptible people.[19] Prevention was a matter of removing decaying matter (early sanitation efforts) and cure frequently entailed removal to some countryside for its purifying airs. And while those sanitation efforts did provide some public health benefit, this was not from understanding the etiology of disease, but lucky happenstance—which ties in to the second thing that should be obvious to any reader: Quarantine is a 650-plus-year-old policy of disease prevention. Why are we relying on a medical practice from the fourteenth century today? We wouldn't use most of 1300s-era medicine, so why this? In the 1300s, knowledge of disease was rudimentary, with limited understanding of why quarantine was effective at all. Broadly applied, we are more knowledgeable now and should act it.

Given that the principle of quarantine is ages old, and the justifications that made it so effective in 1348 are now outdated, we need to reevaluate our therapeutic use of quarantine, taking in to account both theoretical assumptions and actual behavior of people exposed to highly infectious, deadly diseases. If quarantine is to continue being used in contemporary disease management, it should be because there is a valid and contemporary explanation for it, not one whose justification is grounded in beliefs of miasma spreading disease.

The Ethics of Quarantine

Coercive public health interventions are typically justified under the notion that there are times when personal rights such as liberty or autonomy are subsumed to the needs of the community.[20] Childress et al., for example, propose that although there will be conflicts between the moral considerations foundational to their defined goals of modern public health (producing benefits, preventing harms, maximizing utility) and other moral commitments, there is a set of justificatory conditions that will aid in determining whether public health measures may infringe on values such as liberty, equality, justice, and so forth.[21] These five are briefly defined as follows:

Effectiveness: shows that infringing one or more general considerations will probably protect public health (the stated goal of the quarantine must be reachable).

Proportionality: shows that probable public health benefits outweigh the infringed general moral considerations (violations of personal rights must be weighed against positive features such as infection control).

Necessity: there are no other options that can be taken to achieve the public health goal in question (there must be a reason coercion is necessary over any other option).

Least infringement: it minimizes any infringement upon general moral considerations (if you have to step on a moral consideration like privacy, do so with as little intrusion as possible).

Public justification: explaining and justifying the rights infringement.[22]

Now, that stated, it almost immediately becomes clear that the 2013–2016 EVD pandemic fails to meet any of the five necessary justificatory conditions for violating individual rights in favor of the public's health.

Effectiveness. The effectiveness of quarantine was grossly overstated, as seen by the number of people who were confirmed to be infected during their quarantine (in non-pandemic areas, none) versus the number of people quarantined.[23] Even Duncan's fiancée and family, who nursed him while sick and then were quarantined for days in as unsafe a condition as you might be able to dream up, were you inclined to dream scenarios for infecting someone with EVD, did not become infected with EVD.

Proportionality. Quarantine is an out-of-proportion response given that EVD is not contagious until symptomatic; symptoms also appear gradually, so there is time for an infected person to seek medical care before the symptoms become incapacitating—or capable of spreading to other people.

Necessity. There are less restrictive and violating alternatives available, such as symptom monitoring and community health check-in ("surveillance"). Nigeria experienced and successfully contained an outbreak of 20 EVD cases in 2014; among the public health initiatives credited with solving the outbreak were proactive contact tracing and monitoring of exposed individuals. Forced quarantine was not among them.[24]

Least infringing. See above; given the abundance of more effective and less invasive measures, it is not possible for quarantine to be the least infringing public health measure.

Public justification. You can give the public justification for almost anything—but that doesn't mean it is an ethical or moral (let alone good) justification. "Public justification" was fed by Ebolanioa[25] and unscientific, inaccurate fears stoked by many people—often politicians[26]—for political gain in the 2014 American mid-term elections.[27] Because American media dominates international media, said fears spread without justification. Public justification must rely on truthfully representing the effectiveness, proportionality, necessity, and proof that the action being called for is the least restrictive or infringing alternative available. The media is responsible for holding those they are reporting on to those standards.[28] (See Russell in chapter 11.)

Another popular way of evaluating the ethical justification of quarantine is to examine whether it is the least liberty-violating, or least restrictive means,[29] available. However, the reality is that there is no reason liberty should be assumed to be the most important right to preserve.[30] There are situations in which utility, equality, justice, and so forth, might actually be the right we want least violated. Because of this, I reject the phrase "least liberty-violating" or any phraseology that implies we should only care about one value to the exclusion of others; instead, I prefer the phrase "least restrictive option."

This is not terribly pithy and certainly doesn't have the memorable catchiness of "least liberty-violating," but it also does not betray an alliance to any theoretical methodology, and acknowledges that what values are at stake will and likely should change based on the case in front of you. We should not assume that what the least restrictive option is for EVD will be universal, but instead commit to being sensitive to the different properties of infectious diseases.

A False Dilemma

The ethics of quarantine is premised on the apparent dilemma that arises between our obligations to public health and individual rights and liberties. But I contend that this is, in almost all cases, a false dilemma. If one holds to the premise that any coercive social-distancing measure implemented must be proportional to the disease threat, quarantine is *prima facie* impermissible in the case of EVD and other known diseases, because it actively undermines public health efforts.

In order to understand how this can be, it may help to first review the 2002/2003 SARS (Severe Acute Respiratory Syndrome) epidemic, the first modern pandemic to genuinely scare public health and other officials.

In hindsight, the first reported case of SARS occurred in Guangdong Provence, China, in November 2002. Cases spread in China, but the international community was not made aware of any issue until February of 2003. Soon after, the World Health Organization issued a pandemic alert; infections were eventually recorded worldwide.[31]

Limited local transmission of SARS was recorded in fewer places, including Toronto, a city that implemented quarantine during the outbreak. While all of Canada had 440 probable SARS cases, resulting in 40 deaths,[32] approximately 23,000 people in Toronto were quarantined, most confined to their own homes.[33] China quarantined nearly 30,000 people, although nearly sixty percent of those people were detained at centralized quarantine facilities and they had nearly 2,500 probable SARS cases to Toronto's 250.[34]

Of course, the problem in both Toronto and China? Compliance. Stories abound of residents of Amoy Gardens in Hong Kong having fled ahead of officials who came to relocate the entire complex to a quarantine facility,[35] and only 57 percent of those quarantined in Toronto were, according to health authorities, compliant.[36] Although police and public health officials were working together, people were able to evade both if they were so inclined. And in the case of SARS, many were inclined.

While prior to the SARS outbreak, the general belief was that people would be happy to comply with sensible disease requests, like complying with quarantine, the lack of compliance and fleeing from quarantine that happened during SARS should have been an indication of what would come with the 2013–2016 EVD outbreak: People fleeing *cordon sanitaire* and unsanctioned night burials (see Henwood, chapter 2, this volume), evading official quarantine,[37] and the reinforced stigmatization of the ill (see Phelan, chapter 9; and Kruvand, chapter 12, this volume).

Two pandemic outbreaks now show us people resist quarantine measures—and that they are ineffective because of this. The stated goal of quarantine is more effectively achieved via education,[38] monitoring exposed people for signs of the disease,[39] and instituting isolation and treatment should an exposed person start showing signs of infection.

We can thus reach the conclusion that quarantine is of limited use for two reasons: 1) people are noncompliant when faced with quarantine; and 2) it is of limited utility given the equal effectiveness of less restrictive alternatives.[40]

(Ebola) Babies on a Plane: Future Quarantine Scenarios

However, just because the criteria for coerced social distancing via quarantine has not occurred since the dual advent of effective vaccination and antibiotics does not mean that a situation may not occur, at some future time, wherein the Doge of Venice's solution would again be appropriate. While it can be tempting to spin some chaotic tale of a mutant death ferret-flu laboratory escape, in reality, we can utilize a much simpler theoretical case study: a plane full of orphaned newborn infants that were exposed to Ebola virus.[41]

In this scenario, there is a plane full of orphaned newborn infants sitting on an airport tarmac. It is not discovered that they have been exposed to Ebola virus until the plane is airborne; at that time, flight attendants minimize interaction with the infants and the pilots stay inside the cockpit with no direct contact with the passenger cabin. Upon landing, the plane is directed to a distant corner of the airport and the pilots and flight attendants are escorted quickly off the plane and given instructions: They are to monitor themselves for a series of symptoms that indicate EVD, and will be contacted twice a day for 21 days for a status update. This leaves health responders with a quandary: What do they do with these newborn infants, who have no legal guardians to care for them and monitor them for symptoms? Should these babies be released to the lined-up foster or group homes that agreed to take the babies before their infection status was known?

I would argue that, as newborn infants are unable to communicate, a less restrictive alternative to quarantine such as surveillance via daily check-ins would not be possible, and quarantine becomes the most effective and least restrictive public health intervention. Furthermore, disease progression is often an unknown in infants, and while the ongoing EVD outbreak might eventually contribute relevant knowledge for infants and EVD, currently that data is not a part of the literature. An inability to communicate symptomatology and unknown symptom progression of a highly infectious disease seems to result in the argument that quarantine would be the least restrictive alternative for these infants[42] that both provides for their care and also protects the larger community from possible exposure to contagion.

A focus on the science of disease infection, along with the realities of a specific situation on hand, also allows us flexibility in other situations. Currently, Australia quarantines animals that can bring rabies into the country for a 30-day period; animals, much like newborn babies, cannot express symptomatology or express distress in a clear-to-understand manner, and Australia has a vested interest in keeping their island-country rabies-free. A building can be quarantined when exposed to anthrax; buildings cannot communicate illness (yet) and there is no way to know whether or not spores of anthrax remain in the building until a careful and thorough cleaning is done. Fruits, vegetables, and other fauna are subject to border control and quarantine around the world; again, the fact that neither puppies nor potatoes can communicate means that the proportionate response is quarantine.

Conclusion

Mass quarantine is a relic of the past that seems to have largely outlived its usefulness.[43] It is old-fashioned, outdated, and primarily driven by panic and political security theater, actively undermining public health efforts to contain and quell infectious disease spread. In times of infectious disease crises, almost all cases indicate that the least restrictive option available is a watch-and-wait, contact-monitoring surveillance approach, not quarantine. Along with monitoring those exposed to disease for disease-specific symptomology, a mass[44] public education[45] campaign based within the community and on scientific fact, not political elections or ratings, should be implemented.

Childress et al. discuss imposing versus expressing community, which is worthwhile to briefly examine. To impose community is to use the implicit threat of force to gain a desired outcome; for example, coerced social-distancing measures such as quarantine when there are other options available. To express community utilizes solidarity, protects interest, and, importantly, gains trust.[46] An excellent example of this is the multilevel educational and science-communication outreach efforts in the West African nations of Guinea, Sierra Leone, and Liberia.[47] What stopped EVD was a global improvement of health access[48] and knowledge, not quarantine efforts.

The idea that "in a public health emergency there must be a trade-off between effective public health measures and civil rights"[49] tends to be an unquestioned narrative. We are so habituated to the historical narrative of quarantine as a good, no one has stopped to evaluate whether or not it's actually *true* that quarantine is a good. But as Annas notes, "human rights and health are not inherently conflicting goals that must be traded off against each other."[50] In the case of quarantine, the idea that it is the least restrictive option available to control disease outbreak is patently false. The 2013–2016 EVD outbreak shows that, in fact, surveillance is a more effective option to monitor possible infection while also retaining more liberties than quarantine.

A radical reconceptualization of the ethics of quarantine is necessary, and that reaction needs to be disease-sensitive. Different infectious agents have different symptoms and progression, and treating all diseases as alike, capable of being corralled by a single response, is a futile failure of medicine, policy, and rational thought.

Notes

1. Some people split hairs further, discussing soft or voluntary vs. hard or involuntary quarantine. I find this largely unnecessary, since nothing stops people from staying home from their commitments whenever they feel it necessary—and the minute they feel they don't have a choice, it's no longer a voluntary staying home. Whether quarantine is performed at home or in a hospital has little bearing on the fact that it is coerced social distancing.

2. Two other similar and frequently conflated words that are worth knowing the difference between are "contagion" and "infectious." Contagion refers to a disease that is transmissible from person to person and quantified by R-naught, while infectious refers to the number of particles (virions, bacteria, or other pathogens) necessary to infect an exposed individual. See CDC, "Understand Quarantine and Isolation," February 10, 2014, http://www.bt.cdc.gov/preparedness/quarantine/.

3. George Annas, *Worst Case Bioethics* (New York: Oxford University Press, 2010), 226.

4. While it is true that health care workers were attacked, and in some cases killed, attempting to do community outreach in Guinea, Sierra Leone, and Liberia, that has less to do with an unwillingness to receive medical treatment and more with suspicion of certain doctors and government workers. An excellent resource on this is Barry S. Hewlett and Bonnie L. Hewlett, *Ebola, Culture, and Politics: The Anthropology of an Emerging Disease* (Belmont, CA: Thomson Wadsworth, 2007).

5. P. Alcabes, *Dread: How Fear and Fantasy Have Fueled Epidemics from the Black Death to Avian Flu* (Philadelphia: PublicAffairs, 2009), 6.

6. House Energy and Commerce Committee, "Notable Elements of Mr. Duncan's Initial Emergency Department Visit," September 25, 2015, accessed November 1, 2015, http://energycommerce.house.gov/sites/republicans.energycommerce.house.gov/files/Hearings/OI/20141016/Timeline2.pdf.

7. Greg Botelho and Michael Martinez, "Frustrated woman quarantined with sheets, towels soiled by Ebola patient," CNN, October 3, 2014, http://www.cnn.com/2014/10/02/us/texas-woman-quarantine-ebola-thomas-duncan/.

8. F. Karimi, "From Guinea to the U.S.: Timeline of First Ebola patient in New York City," CNN, October 24, 2014, http://www.cnn.com/2014/10/24/health/new-york-ebola-timeline/.

9. S. Spencer, "Having and Fighting Ebola—Public Health Lessons from a Clinician Turned Patient," *The New England Journal of Medicine* 372, 1089–91 (2015), doi: 10.1056/NEJMp1501355.

10. E. Fitzsimmons, "Nurse Who Spoke Out about Quarantine Felt a Calling for Health Care, Friends Say," *The New York Times*, October 26, 2014, http://www.nytimes.com/2014/10/27/nyregion/nurse-who-spoke-out-about-quarantine-felt-a-calling-for-health-care-friends-say.html.

11. K. Hickox, "Her Story: UTA Grad Isolated at New Jersey Hospital in Ebola Quarantine," Dallas Morning News, October 25, 2014, http://www.dallasnews.com/ebola/headlines/20141025-uta-grad-isolated-at-new-jersey-hospital-as-part-of-ebola-quarantine.ece.

12. K. Hickox, "Caught between Civil Liberties and Public Safety Fears: Personal Reflections from a Healthcare Provider Treating Ebola," *Journal of Health and Biomedical Law* 11 (2015): 9–23, http://www.suffolk.edu/documents/LawJournals/Kaci_Hickox_Suffolk_Law_JHBL.pdf.

13. R. S. Gottfried, *The Black Death* (New York: Simon and Schuster, 2010), 48.

14. Perhaps the most famous literary reference would be Apollo sending a plague, via arrow, to the Achaeans in *The Iliad*. While Homer's poem is fictitious, it serves to show that even in approximately 750 BCE, the idea of disease being inflicted as a punishment by the gods was established.

15. However, even at the time where knowledge of disease was not terribly sophisticated, some people understood that there needed to be a distinction between those who were sick and those who merely *might* be sick. The quadrilateral design of the Milanese lazaretto was set up with this in mind: Suspected ill patients are held in one quarter of the hospital; confirmed ill patients are held in a second area; the convalescent in a third; and the fourth area is set aside for hospital staff. Knowing when to move a patient from suspected to confirmed sick to convalescing, though, requires knowledge of disease. Without at least some rudimentary idea of what it looks like to be sick and what it looks like to be well, this sort of separation would be impossible. In other words, knowledge of disease is required before you can determine whether someone is sick.

16. R. Porter, *The Greatest Benefit to Mankind* (New York: W.W. Norton, 1999), 126.

17. Alcabes, *Dread: How Fear and Fantasy Have Fueled Epidemics from the Black Death to Avian Flu,* 42.

18. The most elaborate of these was the *Pestkordon*, running along the Eastern boundary of the Austro-Hungarian Empire. Those traveling west were held, at times for weeks. The effectiveness of this pest-control boundary remains up for debate, especially since the *Pestkordon* itself was completed 15 years after plague left the continent.

19. In fact, this miasmatist theory of disease persisted until the late 1880s, and contributed to the ineffectiveness of the first International Sanitary Conference. See Porter, *The Greatest Benefit to Mankind,* 484.

20. L. O. Gostin, "When Terrorism Threatens Health: How Far Are Limitations on Personal and Economic Liberties Justified?," *Florida Law Review* 55 (2003), 1105; Michael J. Selgelid, "A Moderate Pluralist Approach to Public Health Policy and Ethics," *Public Health Ethics* 2, no. 2 (August 3, 2009): 195–205, doi: 10.1093/phe/php018.

21. James F. Childress, Ruth R. Faden, Ruth D. Gaare, Lawrence Ogalthorpe Gostin, Jeffrey Kahn, Richard J. Bonnie, et al., "Public Health Ethics: Mapping the Terrain," *The Journal of Law, Medicine and Ethics* 30, no. 2 (2002): 170–78.

22. Ibid.

23. This claim applies clearly in the developed world; in the developing world, independent of what we might think about effectiveness given a higher incidence, there are other reasons to doubt the overall effectiveness of quarantine.

24. Alexandra Sifferlin, "Nigeria is Ebola-Free: Here's What They Did Right," *TIME,* October 19, 2014, http://time.com/3522984/ebola-nigeria-who/.

25. "Ebolanoia" was coined by science journalist Maryn McKenna in October 2014 to express people's irrational fear of contracting Ebola in countries that were not experiencing Ebola outbreaks.

26. W. Engelhardt, "How ISIS and Ebola Took over the Midterm Elections," *Mother Jones,* November 14, 2014, http://www.motherjones.com/politics/2014/11/how-isis-and-ebola-took-over-midterm-elections.

27. T. Barrett and Deidre Walsh, "Ebola becomes an election issue," CNN, October 3, 2014, http://www.cnn.com/2014/10/03/politics/ebola-midterms/.

28. M. Gertz and Rob Savillo, "Report: Ebola Coverage on TV News Plummeted after Midterms," *Media Matters,* November 19, 2014, http://mediamatters.org/research/2014/11/19/report-ebola-coverage-on-tv-news-plummeted-afte/201619.

29. A full discussion of the conflicting values of liberty, utility, and equality is available in Selgelid, "A Modern Pluralist Approach to Public Health Policy and Ethics."

30. Selgelid, "A Modern Pluralist Approach to Public Health Policy and Ethics"; Childress et al., "Public Health Ethics: Mapping the Terrain."

31. Institute of Medicine, "Learning from SARS: Preparing for the Next Disease Outbreak: Workshop Summary," 2004, http://www.ncbi.nlm.nih.gov/books/NBK92478/.

32. L. K. Altman, "Fearing SARS, Ontario Urges Wider Quarantines," *New York Times,* April 18, 2003.

33. This was dubbed "sheltering in place," a term many will recall is more frequently associated with bioterrorism attacks. The overlap in language is not a coincidence, as the securitization of public health has been intentional since the 2001 American anthrax "Amerithrax" attacks and subsequent Biomedical Advanced Research and Development Authority funding.

34. M. Rothstein, M. Gabriela Alcalde, Nanette R. Elster, Mary Anderlik Majumder, Larry I. Palmer, T. Howard Stone, et al. "Quarantine and Isolation: Lessons Learned from SARS, A Report to the Centers for Disease Control and Prevention," November 2003, http://www.iaclea.org/members/pdfs/SARS%20REPORT.Rothstein.pdf.

35. M. Pottinger, et al. "Quarantine Quandary," *Wall Street Journal*, April 1, 2003.

36. T. Svoboda, B. Henry, L. Shulman, E. Kennedy, E. Rea, W. Ng, et al., "Public Health Measures to Control the Spread of Severe Acute Respiratory Syndrome during the Outbreak in Toronto," *The New England Journal of Medicine* 350 (2004): 2352–61.

37. D. Henshaw, "In Liberia, Burial Practices Hinder Battle Against Ebola," *Wall Street Journal*, September 1, 2014, http://www.wsj.com/articles/in-liberia-burial-practices-hinder-battle-against-ebola-1409619832.

38. G. York, "Fear and Education Play a Crucial Role in Ebola Crisis," *The Globe and Mail*, October 9, 2014, http://www.theglobeandmail.com/life/health-and-fitness/health/fear-and-education-play-crucial-role-in-ebola-crisis/article20999262/.

39. Self-monitoring and frequent contact, often by cell phones, is how Nigeria managed to quickly contain their arm of the ongoing Ebola outbreak. See Elahe Izadi, "What Texas Can Learn from Nigeria When It Comes to Containing Ebola," *Washington Post*, October 4, 2014, https://www.washingtonpost.com/news/to-your-health/wp/2014/10/04/what-texas-can-learn-from-nigeria-when-it-comes-to-containing-ebola/?Post+generic=%3Ftid%3Dsm_twitter_washingtonpost.

40. It is common to discuss quarantine in terms of least-liberty violating, but this makes a mistake in placing a perhaps unconscious emphasis on a single right within its phrasing: liberty. However, the reality, as Selgelid and Childress et al. have noted separately, is that there is no reason liberty should be assumed the most important right to preserve. There are situations in which utility, equality, justice, and so forth, might actually be the right we want least violated—hence opting instead for the phrase least rights restricting; regardless of the right in play, the option selected should be that which least restricts that right. While "least liberty-violating" is quippy and memorable, it would behoove us to remember accuracy over infectious phrasing. See Selgelid, "A Moderate Pluralist Perspective on Public Health Ethics," and Childress et al., "Public Health Ethics: Mapping the Terrain."

41. I acknowledge that thought experiments are often considered the bane of philosophical dialogue—a belief I cheerfully advocated until the advent of self-driving cars and the sudden, immediate relevance of Judith Jarvis Thomson's seminal work

with the trolley problem. See e.g., P. Lin, "The Ethics of Autonomous Cars," *The Atlantic,* October 8, 2013, http://www.theatlantic.com/technology/archive/2013/10/the-ethics-of-autonomous-cars/280360/. In reality, a well-described thought experiment should help us to isolate and define the key variables under examination, test our assumptions, and either confirm or refute theoretical claims. Whether "Ebola babies on a plane" succeeds is a determination I will leave to the reader.

42. Some scholars might be tempted to argue that infants do not have full moral agency. While I would likely find this argument *compelling,* for this paper I don't feel that it is *necessary.* Whether an infant is a moral agent is immaterial to facts we can all agree on: Infants cannot effectively communicate any symptoms they are experiencing to their caregiver, save crying. While an effective strategy to indicate distress, it is not one that can differentiate between needing a nappy change and the joint aches and pains that accompany EVD. See, e.g., Mary Anne Warren, *Moral Status: Obligations to Persons and Other Living Things* (Clarendon Press, 2000).

43. Annas, *Worst Case Bioethics,* 227.

44. J. Poole, "'Shadow' and 'D-12' Sing An Infectious Song About Ebola," NPR, August 19, 2014, http://www.npr.org/sections/goatsandsoda/2014/08/19/341412011/shadow-and-d-12-sing-an-infectious-song-about-ebola.

45. S. Jones, "African musicians band together to raise Ebola awareness," *The Guardian,* October 29, 2014, http://www.theguardian.com/global-development/2014/oct/29/african-musicians-record-song-ebola-awareness.

46. Childress et al., "Public Health Ethics: Mapping the Terrain."

47. J. Beaubien, "Liberian Singers Use the Power of Music to Raise Ebola Awareness," NPR, October 12, 2014, http://www.npr.org/2014/10/12/355427316/liberian-singers-use-the-power-of-music-to-raise-ebola-awareness.

48. Selgelid, "A Moderate Pluralist Perspective on Public Health Ethics."

49. James F. Childress and Ruth Gaare Bernheim, "Beyond the Liberal and Communitarian Impasse: A Framework and Vision for Public Health," *Florida Law Review,* 55 (2003): 1191.

50. G. J. Annas, "Bioterrorism, Public Health, and Human Rights," *Health Affairs* 21, no. 6 (November 2002): 94–97.

Epilogue: Ethical Lessons from Ebola Virus Disease

Lisa M. Lee

Nulla (enim) res tantum ad dicendum proficit, quantum scriptio.
—Cicero

Nothing so much assists learning as writing down what we wish to remember. Reflecting on Cicero's words and all of those written in this book, there is much to remember—and much to learn—from the 2013–2016 West African Ebola virus disease (EVD) epidemic. This chapter summarizes the deliberations and recommendations of the Presidential Commission for the Study of Bioethical Issues (Bioethics Commission) as outlined in its February 2015 report, *Ethics and Ebola: Public Health Planning and Response.* The Bioethics Commission examined the ethical dimensions of the ongoing epidemic and wrote down what it wished for us to remember as we face future public health emergencies. In the report, the Bioethics Commission observed, "The current Ebola epidemic reveals how our engagement in outbreaks of infectious disease can reflect national values. Deliberate development of public health policies in accordance with high ethical and evidentiary standards is the mark of a society committed to national and global health."[1] This sentiment forms the basis of the Bioethics Commission's seven recommendations for future public health preparedness planning.

The Ethical and Prudential Imperative to Act

Although slow to react during the first half of the Ebola epidemic, international response grew throughout late 2014 and early 2015. Once cases of EVD were diagnosed outside the western African region, governments—including officials in the United States—came to realize that engagement in this global public health emergency served the collective interests of all nations. Stemming the tide of infection at its source, preventing global spread, and stabilizing political and economic systems at risk of collapse from the devastating outbreak represented important pragmatic and self-interested motivations for global action. Engagement based on such enlightened self-interest and recognition that our interests are interconnected and mutually reinforcing have the potential to move us toward a wider worldview that incorporates a moral imperative.

The West ultimately recognized that it had a moral imperative, based in our common humanity, to provide assistance in the face of abject suffering. Both the public and those in a professional position to respond recognized the great need for engagement. Whether based in social justice and the obligation to respond to the health needs of the severely disadvantaged, or in the tacit expectations resulting from former colonial relationships, the ethical justification for intervention was clear.

In the end, the West's response revealed both its ethical and prudential interests in fighting Ebola, even if half a world away. In its first recommendation, the Bioethics Commission concluded, "In an interconnected world, for ethical reasons and to protect national interests, the US government has a responsibility to engage in preparedness and to participate in coordinated global responses to public health emergencies."[2]

Further noting that an effective public health response to future emergencies requires coordinated public health infrastructure and international response capacity, the Bioethics Commission's second recommendation was to strengthen key elements of the United States's global response capabilities. Specific measures cited for improvement included strengthening the World Health Organization through increased funding and collaboration with other governmental and nongovernmental responders; empowering a single US health official to serve as the responsible party for all federal response to domestic and international public health emergencies; and strengthening the deployment capability of the US Public Health Service, which serves as the US point organization for public health emergency response.[3]

In the face of a public health emergency, public support for domestic policy and global engagement requires transparency and accountability. Engaging the public through clear communication of scientifically sound information—as well as recognizing and acknowledging existing uncertainties—fosters trust and support for action in response to public health emergencies. In chapter 8 of this volume, Kim Yi Dionne and Laura Seay describe the multiple misconceptions held by the American public during the 2013–2016 EVD epidemic.[4] As they report, misperceptions about geography and history can have devastating effects in a global public health emergency.

Clear information about how population health during an outbreak differs from individual clinical care, for example, can assist the public with understanding the need for movement restrictions and other effective public health interventions such as contact tracing. Evidence-based policies that reduce—or at least do not exacerbate—existing inequities are critical. In addition, policies based on the least possible infringement of personal liberty are ethically preferable. If choosing between policy options, all else being equal, the one with the least intrusion on individual freedom is the most defensible choice.

Preparation for public health emergencies includes not only planning logistics and ensuring necessary supplies, but also preparing the public. Proactive deliberation and education before emergencies can assist public officials with addressing conflicting values that can complicate policy making in our diverse society. Deliberative decision making requires time. It involves exploration of a plurality of views, reflection, and respectful exchange of ideas. Engaging in deliberative processes as a part of public health preparedness is best begun during non-emergent times. Inevitably, public engagement is necessary during emergencies as well, and public health should put these systems in place during nonemergency deliberations for use during or in the aftermath of crises.

Effective communication is directly connected to successful uptake of public health policies, and the Bioethics Commission recommended that public health professionals educate the public and communicate clearly about the nature and justification of public health responses. Communication efforts should provide the public with accurate information about the response, including what is known and what is not known. Efforts also must provide persons most directly affected by public health response policies with the reasoning behind them, as well as the values reflected in policy implementation. Across all communication efforts, the Bioethics Commission urged approaches and techniques that mitigate stigmatization and discrimination that can result during public health emergencies.[5]

One of the most poignant lessons from this Ebola outbreak was the need for real-time integration of ethical decision making to complement response planning. The Bioethics Commission noted that during public health emergencies, public health professionals and policymakers need responsive and accessible resources to assist them with the myriad ethical challenges that inevitably arise in the course of the response. Patricia Henwood remarks on the need for "real-time evolution" of EVD management in chapter 2.[6] Integration of ethics into this real-time evolution is essential in order to facilitate questions of what we *should* do that are raised by emerging questions of what we *can* do. These ethical problem-solving resources work best when they are integrated into the established public health infrastructure. While calling in a consulting ethicist when something troubling arises in the midst of a crisis can be helpful, policy decisions that incorporate ethical considerations during the planning process can help public health professionals anticipate, identify, and address ethical concerns throughout policy development and implementation. Including ethical expertise in response monitoring and post-response evaluations also can assist with preparation for future emergencies.

To ensure that ethical principles are incorporated into timely and agile public health emergency response, the Bioethics Commission recommended, "Qualified public health ethics expertise should be readily available to identify ethical considerations relevant to public health emergencies and responses in light of real-time available evidence."[7] To realize ethics integration as more than an add-on from outside the public health infrastructure, the commission recommended that a single US public health official be accountable for all domestic and international emergency response, including integrating ethics as an essential part of the response.[8]

Public Health Practice and Research during Emergencies

In the 2013–2016 EVD epidemic, several US public health actions required thorough ethical consideration. The lack of ethics engagement in planning for such an emergency led to real-time examination of three especially challenging issues: quarantine, the use of placebo-controlled trials, and the collection and sharing of biospecimens.

Quarantine

From a public health practice perspective, requiring and enforcing movement restrictions during an infectious disease outbreak raises a number of ethical considerations, many of which are outlined by Kelly Hills in chapter 16.[9] Most of these challenges revolve around the tension between the individual liberty we have come to expect in liberal democracies and the communal orientation of public health interventions needed to contain the spread of disease. Limiting one's ability to move about and interact freely is a severe intervention and ought be applied only when nothing less will serve the same end. This claim is based on the principle of least infringement, which requires public health officials to implement the least intrusive approach to achieve the public health goal. What measures achieve the public health goal depend on characteristics of the infectious agent as well as willingness of affected communities to participate. Agent characteristics include mode and ease of transmission, the infectious period, severity of resulting illness, availability of treatment, and associated mortality, among others. Community willingness to abide by public health movement restrictions depends on a clear understanding of and justification for such measures. Affected communities must be assured that the policy is evidence-based, represents the least possible infringement on individual liberty for the shortest duration, and is implemented justly and equitably.

The Bioethics Commission examined lessons from past epidemics such as SARS, tuberculosis, and HIV. During the 2002–2003 SARS epidemic, countries across the globe experienced various levels of cooperation with quarantine and isolation orders. Success was correlated with vigorous public education and financial subsidies for missed wages and other expenses for persons quarantined. Tuberculosis, like SARS, is spread via respiratory droplets expelled when an infectious persons sneezes or coughs. Public health laws in US states give public health officials authority to quarantine and isolate infectious persons, but these restrictive orders are enforced only after less intrusive measures, such as directly observed therapy, fail. HIV, unlike SARS and tuberculosis, is relatively difficult to transmit; it requires contact with infected blood, semen, or vaginal fluid. Still, for the first few decades of the epidemic, fear drove much of the public response and many policy decisions. The need for accurate communication of evidence-based information remains in the fight against HIV and other infectious pathogens. A lesson common to all of these examples is the need to anticipate and mitigate public fear. When an infectious threat creates fear—real or imagined—communities often marginalize and stigmatize persons whom they perceive to be a threat. This "othering" often has severe social consequences ranging from discrimination to property damage to physical harm or death in egregious cases, as Kim Yi Dionne and Laura Seay discuss in chapter 8. Unfortunately, these consequences still occur. In the 2013–2016 EVD epidemic, Liberian-Americans and other members of the African diaspora reported experiencing overt hostility from strangers. Health care workers returning from volunteering in western Africa faced discrimination themselves and worried that their families would suffer consequences by association. These experiences give us an opportunity to consider carefully what ethical dimensions must be addressed when considering movement restrictions.

The Bioethics Commission outlined five ethical principles or conditions that provide justification for movement restrictions in the face of a public health emergency. The first two, the harm principle and the principle of least infringement, address the importance of minimizing the impingement on individual liberty. The harm principle guides us to limit the restrictions on individual liberty to those necessary to keep an individual or group from harming others. The principle of least infringement supports the imposition of the least intrusive effective public health interventions; if another intervention is as effective, but intrudes less on liberty, it should be used in place of the more intrusive one. The third principle, beneficence, along with its corollary, nonmaleficence, guides us to consider interventions that promote benefit while not introducing harm. Movement restriction in the context of an infectious disease epidemic can promote great benefit, but is not without harms. In this case, a related concept, proportionality, requires that the probable benefit of the intervention is sufficient to justify its burden. The fourth principle, reciprocity, compels us to consider necessary support for persons who bear the burden of interventions that protect the public's health. Examples of reciprocal support include access to goods such as food and clothing, compensation for lost income, and protection and care for dependents. Specific types and amount of support are determined by context and depend, in part, on the size of the affected population. Finally, the commission included justice and fairness as an essential ethical consideration for movement restriction.

This principle requires that the benefits and burdens of public health response be distributed equitably and not exacerbate existing disparities. For example, discriminatory practices such as imposing restrictions on whole subsets of the population without evidence-based justification are unjust.

These principles are reflected in the Bioethics Commission's fifth recommendation, which states, "Governments and public health organizations should employ the least restrictive means necessary—on the basis of the best available scientific evidence—in implementing restrictive public health measures, such as quarantines and travel restrictions."[10] The commission concludes this recommendation stating that public health officials have an ethical duty to clearly communicate the rationale for restrictive measures, especially to persons most affected by them, and to update related requirements as evidence develops.

Public Health Research

The conduct of public health and clinical research during an emergency raises numerous ethical questions. Whether research should be done at all when care needs are high is less controversial than exactly how such research ought to be conducted. Annette Rid describes some of the ethical debate associated with conducting research during the 2013–2016 epidemic in chapter 14.[11]

In its ethical analysis the Bioethics Commission recognized an ethical obligation to learn what we can in the presence of a public health emergency in order to provide the best possible management of the situation, and—importantly—to prepare for the next emergency. There are numerous challenges to conducting research ethically in the midst of a public health emergency, including incorporating rapidly changing information; ensuring resources are used to attend to urgent health and safety needs; and ensuring just and equitable distribution of benefits. Research can only go forward on a foundation of public trust. This trust must be built during non-emergency times and maintained in the midst of a crisis. Morenike Oluwatoyin Folayan and Bridget Haire describe the importance of community trust in chapter 15.[12] Proactive public deliberation and transparency are keys to coping with communities in great need. Building capacity for public engagement of affected persons and their families, communities, and leaders is as essential as conducing first-rate science.

Placebo-Controlled Trials

One of the two predominant research ethics-related issues raised during the early months of the 2013–2016 Ebola epidemic was the use of placebos in clinical testing of pharmaceutical treatments and vaccine candidates. With no known treatment and no effective vaccine in the face of a lethal virus, trials to develop these were sorely needed. The placebo-controlled trial is the most scientifically rigorous way to show effectiveness of a drug candidate, producing results with the fewest participants in the shortest time compared with other methods. However, such trials require that some participants be randomly assigned to receive a "sugar pill" or inactive dose of the trial medication. This produces an ethical tension between speed of discovery and the reality that, in public health emergencies involving such high mortality rates, all persons want access to medicines with even a remote possibility of helping.

Researchers have been debating the ethics of the use of placebos in clinical trials for many years. Withholding treatment to test the safety and efficacy of a new intervention is ethically complex. However, in a situation like the Ebola epidemic where there are no approved treatments, the ethical argument is not whether to withhold existing treatment, but rather whether or not all patients should be given a treatment that has the possibility of benefit, even if the benefit is unproven and the treatment could cause harm. Requiring the best possible research design, given the constraints and the context, is morally required. The Bioethics Commission has held that ethical science begins with quality science.[13] Undertaking flawed science lacks social value and puts participants at risk while yielding no possibility of societal benefit.

The Bioethics Commission considered four ethically relevant considerations for examining the ethical challenges involved in choosing a research design that provides the best possible evidence in the shortest period (i.e., a placebo-controlled trial) and other designs that would provide all participants with potential benefit but might take longer, require more participants, or possibly compromise interpretation of results. First, there are important scientific and ethical differences between vaccine trials and treatment trials. In vaccine trials, participants are healthy volunteers and are not likely to directly benefit from participation. In vaccine trials, it is ethically preferable to include as few healthy volunteers as possible to achieve accurate scientific results—again, through the placebo-controlled trial.

Second, when considering a disease like Ebola, where mortality is high and there are no known treatments, treatment trials by definition include persons who are ill and in need of supportive care. In a placebo-controlled trial design, participants should receive the best available supportive care. The definition of "best available supportive care" must be addressed. Does it mean the best *possible* care available anywhere? The best possible care given the circumstances? The level and type of care that is sustainable in the local context once the research is complete? Providing sustainable supportive care is most prudent for numerous reasons, two of which include longer-term sustainability once international aid retreats and ensuring that superior supportive care in a treatment trial does not mask results of an effective treatment.

Third, the Bioethics Commission considered the important role of community responsiveness in designing effective trials. Affected persons must be willing to participate in clinical trials, which makes it critical to engage communities about what is palatable with respect to research design. The best trial design is rendered useless if communities are unwilling to participate in the study.

Lastly, considering their contention that ethical science begins with good science, the Bioethics Commission considered that while differences remain between persons advocating for placebo-controlled trials and those arguing for alternative designs, the primary concern is that the trial design yield credible results. Risks to participants cannot be justified if trial design does not allow for benefit to be realized.

Consideration of these factors led the Bioethics Commission to its sixth recommendation stating that research should be designed to ensure that all participants receive the best supportive care that is sustainably available in the host community. Researchers should implement methodologically rigorous designs that produce clearly interpretable results and are acceptable to the host community. Carefully designed placebo-controlled trials can meet these demands; where they cannot, innovative designs such as adaptive randomized trials should be considered. Research teams should engage with affected communities to determine what trial design best meets the extant ethical and scientific requirements.[14]

Collection and Future Use of Biospecimens

Another research-related concern that garnered attention during this Ebola epidemic was the ethical collection and future use of biospecimens for research. Like the placebo issue, the collection and future use of biospecimens is not unique to the Ebola epidemic. The literature on this topic is robust, and the Bioethics Commission first addressed it in their report, *Privacy and Progress in Whole Genome Sequencing.*[15] Familiar ethical considerations like privacy and consent exist in the public health emergency context as well, but there are additional ethical complexities to which researchers must attend in an infectious disease outbreak and potential pandemic in low- and middle-income countries. One of these concerns equitable benefit sharing. Animated by reciprocity and justice, persons and communities that provide samples must not be denied access to the benefits derived from them. This concern is especially important when the specimens must be transported to high-resource laboratories equipped to perform research with dangerous pathogens, which generally exist in more developed countries. Allowing specimens to be collected and used for research requires trust that the benefits will be available to the communities that supplied the biospecimens, even if that community cannot afford to purchase them at market value. As the opportunity to acquire specimens might arise only during a public health emergency, researchers and policymakers would benefit from engaging with global partners in planning for biospecimen collection.

In the last recommendation in *Ethics and Ebola*, the Bioethics Commission called on the US government and global partners to ensure that biospecimens are obtained ethically and to facilitate access to the resulting benefits to the broadest group possible. They recommended that global partners "work collaboratively with local scientists whenever possible to develop effective strategies for ensuring equitable distribution of the benefits of research."[16]

Conclusion

While not officially declared over, as of September 2015 the epidemic had waned considerably, and Sierra Leone, Guinea, and Liberia had begun to rebuild. Schools were back in session after closure for nearly an entire academic year; care once again was available from antenatal clinics, which were closed to accommodate Ebola patients and to avoid spreading the disease. Before the lens of history colors our memory, we are right to ensure that the lessons of the largest, most widespread Ebola virus epidemic in history guide our public health planning and response. It is clear that a swift, evidence-based response to public health emergencies is ethically required and prudentially justified. Our public health preparedness includes ethical preparedness, and we are wise to ensure early and explicit infusion of ethical considerations and problem solving into our public health emergency response.

Disclaimer

The content of this manuscript represents the opinions and conclusions of the author and does not necessarily represent those of the US Presidential Commission for the Study of Bioethical Issues or the US Department of Health and Human Services.

Notes

1. Presidential Commission for the Study of Bioethical Issues, *Ethics and Ebola: Public Health Planning and Response* (Presidential Commission for the Study of Bioethical Issues: Washington, DC, 2015), 3.

2. Ibid., Recommendation 1, 16.

3. Ibid., Recommendation 2, 17.

4. K. Y. Dionne and L. Seay, "American Perceptions of Africa during an Ebola Outbreak," chapter 8, this volume.

5. Presidential Commission for the Study of Bioethical Issues, *Ethics and Ebola: Public Health Planning and Response,* Recommendation 3, 19.

6. P. Henwood, "Ebola in West Africa: From the Frontline," chapter 2, this volume.

7. Presidential Commission for the Study of Bioethical Issues, *Ethics and Ebola: Public Health Planning and Response,* Recommendation 4, 20.

8. Ibid.

9. K. E. Hills, "Quarantine and Ebola," chapter 16, this volume.

10. Presidential Commission for the Study of Bioethical Issues, *Ethics and Ebola: Public Health Planning and Response,* Recommendation 5, 31.

11. A. Rid, "(How) Should Experimental Vaccines and Treatments for Ebola Be Used?," chapter 14, this volume.

12. M. O. Folayan and B. Haire, "History, Culture, and Social Norms: Implications for Ebola Drug Clinical Trials in Affected Regions," chapter 15, this volume.

13. Presidential Commission for the Study of Bioethical Issues, *Moral Science: Protecting Participants in Human Subjects Research* (Washington, DC: Presidential Commission for the Study of Bioethical Issues, 2011), 90.

14. Presidential Commission for the Study of Bioethical Issues, *Ethics and Ebola: Public Health Planning and Response,* Recommendation 6, p. 42.

15. Presidential Commission for the Study of Bioethical Issues, *Privacy and Progress in Whole Genome Sequencing* (Washington, DC: Presidential Commission for the Study of Bioethical Issues, 2012).

16. Presidential Commission for the Study of Bioethical Issues, *Ethics and Ebola: Public Health Planning and Response,* Recommendation 7, p. 50.

About the Authors

Christian L. Althaus studied biology at ETH Zurich, Switzerland, and obtained a PhD in theoretical biology at Utrecht University, The Netherlands. He is currently leading a research group in immunoepidemiology at the Institute of Social and Preventive Medicine at the University of Bern, Switzerland. His research focuses on better understanding how infectious diseases respond to changes in their environment. For example, he studies how changes in human behavior, vaccination, or drug treatment can affect the prevalence of various infections. In September 2014, Dr. Althaus published the first estimates of the basic reproduction number R_0 of EVD in Guinea, Sierra Leone, and Liberia. This study was of paramount importance in highlighting the lack in controlling the outbreak in Liberia, and was later confirmed by the World Health Organization and several other research groups. During the MERS-CoV outbreak in South Korea from May to July 2015, his research group provided real-time estimates of the reproduction number and published a timely study on the role of superspreading events for newly observed MERS-CoV clusters. More information about Dr. Althaus' work can be found on his research group website (http://www.immuno-epidemiology.ch). He frequently uses Twitter (@c_althaus) to communicate his latest findings and engage in scientific discussions.

Daniel G. Bausch is an Associate Professor in the Department of Tropical Medicine at Tulane School of Public Health and Tropical Medicine and also serves as the Technical Lead for the Epidemic Clinical Management Team in the Pandemic and Epidemic Diseases Department of the World Health Organization, Geneva, Switzerland. Dr. Bausch specializes in the research and control of emerging tropical viruses, with over 20 years' experience in sub-Saharan Africa, Latin America, and Asia combating viruses such as Ebola, Lassa, hantavirus, and SARS coronavirus. He has been extensively involved in the 2013–2016 Ebola virus outbreak in West Africa, working to organize and provide patient care, promote and conduct applied research on Ebola virus, develop guidelines and spur innovation on appropriate personal protective equipment, and advise on the use of experimental therapies and vaccines. Dr. Bausch is the Scientific Program Chair of the American Society of Tropical Medicine and Hygiene. He places a strong emphasis on capacity building in all his projects and also has a keen interest in the role of the scientist in promoting health and human rights.

Adia Benton is an assistant professor of anthropology and African studies at Northwestern University. A social anthropologist who studies the political economy and moral worlds of biomedicine and public health, she writes about infectious diseases, global disparities in access to surgery, and the ideologies of global health and development aid. Her first book, *HIV Exceptionalism: Development through Disease in Sierra Leone,* was published by the University of Minnesota Press in 2015 and describes the global HIV/AIDS industry through a case study of HIV support groups in Freetown, Sierra Leone. Before becoming a professor, she worked as a consultant to numerous aid agencies on development and health throughout the world. She tweets about politics, anthropology, and popular culture from @ethnography911 and blogs anthropological "takes" on current events at http://ethnography911.org.

Michael J. Connor, Jr., MD, is an assistant professor of medicine at Emory University School of Medicine, where he specializes in adult critical care medicine and nephrology. He is an internationally recognized expert in volume management and hemodynamic support in the critically ill, acute kidney injury, renal replacement therapy in the critically ill, and antibiotic therapy during renal replacement therapy. In September 2014, Dr. Connor spearheaded the first-ever application of advanced critical care support to a patient with Ebola virus disease that included the first known successful treatment with acute continuous hemodialysis and mechanical ventilation.

Kim Yi Dionne is assistant professor of government at Smith College. She studies health interventions, politics, and public opinion, primarily in

African countries. She is also a co-contributing editor for Africa content at The Monkey Cage, a blog on politics and political science at the *Washington Post* (https://www.washingtonpost.com/news/monkey-cage/). Her research has been published in *Health Politics and Policy, World Development,* and *Comparative Political Studies*, among other journals and edited volumes. She is on Twitter at @dadakim.

Nicholas G. Evans is an Assistant Professor in Philosophy at the University of Massachusetts Lowell. In 2015 he held an Emerging Leaders in Biosecurity Initiative Fellowship at the UPMC Center for Health Security and a postdoctoral fellowship in advanced biomedical ethics at the Department of Medical Ethics and Health Policy in the Perelman School of Medicine, University of Pennsylvania, during which the bulk of the work for *Ebola's Message* was completed. Dr. Evans conducts research on the security aspects of microbiology and infectious diseases, with a focus on dual-use virology research of concern. He has published work in bioethics in *The Journal of Medical Ethics, mBio, Science and Engineering Ethics,* and *Law and Biosciences.* He also maintains an active research program in military ethics; his first volume, *The Routledge Handbook of Ethics and War*, was released in 2013. He can be found on Twitter at @neva9257.

Morenike Oluwatoyin Folayan holds a fellowship at the West African College of Surgeons as well as a master of business administration. She works in the HIV prevention field building capacity to enable communities to engage effectively in HIV prevention research, and addressing the ethics of community engagement in research. She is currently an associate professor in the Department of Child Dental Health at Obafemi Awolowo University, Ile-Ife; coordinates the Health Sciences and Professional Education Unit of the Institute of Public Health; and is the chair of the Research Innovation and Support Unit and the deputy director of the College of Health Sciences Research and Partnership Advancement Unit at Obafemi Awolowo University. She also coordinates the New HIV Vaccine and Microbicide Advocacy Society.

Stephen Goldstein is a doctoral candidate in cell and molecular biology at the University of Pennsylvania in the laboratory of Susan R. Weiss. He is currently studying Middle Eastern respiratory syndrome coronavirus (MERS-CoV) accessory proteins and working to establish an in vitro model of bat coronavirus infection in the natural host. His interest in Ebola virus dates back to reading the *Hot Zone* in the late 1990s, and he has been deeply involved in online coverage and discussion of the West Africa Ebola virus epidemic. Previously, he received a BA in international affairs at George Washington University and an MS in molecular microbiology and immunology at the Johns Hopkins University Bloomberg School of Public Health in the laboratory of Diane E. Griffin, where he studied the innate immune response to alphavirus infection of neurons. When not doing research, he is most likely to be found skiing in Vermont, British Columbia, or Colorado. He can be found tweeting about both viruses and skiing @stgoldst.

Bridget Haire is a postdoctoral research fellow at the Kirby Institute, University of New South Wales (UNSW) Australia, and president of the Australian Federation of AIDS Organisations, the federation for the community-based response to HIV in Australia. She has published in the areas of research ethics, public health, and human rights, particularly with regard to HIV and other bloodborne infections, sexual health, and Ebola. Her academic work has included lecturing in public health and medical ethics at UNSW, and bioethics and medical humanities at the University of Sydney. Bridget has a strong commitment to community-based responses and has worked in HIV and sexual and reproductive health for 21 years as a journalist, editor, policy analyst, and advocate. She is a consultant for the Australia-China Human Rights Technical Cooperation Program on sexual and reproductive health rights for the Australian Human Rights Commission and serves on the Global Emerging Pathogens consortium and the New South Wales Assessment Panel for the Management of People with HIV Who Risk Infecting Others. She was the medical ethicist on the Data Safety Monitoring Board for the South African HIV prevention study CAPRISA 008. She holds a masters of bioethics and a PhD in standards of care in HIV prevention research.

Patricia C. Henwood, MD, is an Instructor in Emergency Medicine at Harvard Medical School and works clinically as an emergency physician with a focus on point-of-care ultrasound training and research in the emergency, developing world, and disaster contexts. Dr. Henwood worked clinically in two Ebola treatment units in Liberia during the Ebola epidemic in 2014 and 2015. She is now involved in post-Ebola health system strengthening efforts in Liberia. Dr. Henwood has worked in the global health arena for more than a decade, and in 2011 she co-founded Point-of-care Ultrasound in Resource-limited Environments (PURE; www.pureultrasound.org). PURE is dedicated to enhancing ultrasound use, training, and research in resource-limited settings. PURE currently runs ultrasound training programs at national referral hospitals in Liberia, Uganda, and Rwanda. Dr. Henwood serves as PURE's president and has received numerous grants and awards for her research and training in this area. Dr. Henwood attended Georgetown University and Jefferson Medical College. She completed her medical training at the Harvard-affiliated Emergency Medicine Residency at Massachusetts General Hospital and Brigham and Women's Hospital, where she served as chief resident. She completed a fellowship in emergency ultrasound at Brigham and Women's Hospital, where she currently works as an attending emergency medicine physician.

Kelly Hills is a science writer and editor currently living and working in the suburbs of Philadelphia. Prior to this detour, Kelly was a doctoral student in a now-defunct joint degree program in bioethics and philosophy. During that time, she was an in-demand blogger for several bioethics-focused websites. Kelly relocated to the East Coast from Seattle, where she completed her undergraduate degree at the University of Washington in the program on Comparative History of Ideas and the Department of Medical History and Ethics, which means she's excellent at Trivial Pursuit and prone to bouts of Continental philosophy when tired. She's apparently supposed to note that she was inducted into Phi Beta Kappa while there, and graduated with honors and confetti. She also wrote a popular weekly column on bioethics and pop culture; one of the best compliments she ever received was having an article used as a dartboard by an angry pharmacy school. Back in ancient history, Kelly worked in the software industry as a test engineer, where she was known for being able to break anything inside 15 minutes. Kelly's current areas of interest include power and harassment, accountability in biosecurity, biosafety, trust, and sneaking back into graduate school. She lives in a run-down Victorian house with her three cats (Toledo, Overlord Zeus, and Princess Harley); her international partner in crime (also known as "her husband"); and, in the summer, swarms of fireflies, all of whom are named Kaylee. You can find Kelly on social media at @rocza, or occasionally blogging at http://www.kellyhills.com/blog.

Cyril Ibe, a Nigerian-born journalist, has been teaching journalism and digital media at Central State University, Wilberforce, Ohio, since 2006. Ibe is digital content producer for the National Association of African Journalists, a U.S.-based organization of African-born journalists in the diaspora. He was co-founder and managing editor of the now-defunct Chicago-based *African Newbreed*. He has worked as a staff writer for Pioneer Press Newspapers in Chicago and as a general assignment intern reporter at the *Cincinnati Enquirer* and former *Pittsburgh Press*. Ibe has contributed to several other print and online publications, including the *Dayton Weekly News* and All Digitocracy. Ibe was host and executive producer of *Miami Valley Journal*, an hour-long public affairs program on the Central State University public radio station. He has been an invited facilitator of college radio workshops for multimedia journalism classes at Allegheny College in Meadville, Pennsylvania. Ibe also taught as an adjunct professor of media studies at Wilberforce University, Wilberforce, Ohio, and was an adjunct professor of communications, media arts, and theater at Chicago State University in 2000 and a 1999 fellow in the Pew Charitable Trusts' International Reporting Project. Ibe earned a bachelor's degree in communications from Central State University and a master's degree in journalism from Ohio University in Athens, Ohio. Ibe is a doctoral student in health sciences (global health educator/researcher) at Trident University in Cypress, California. Follow him on Twitter @cyrilibe.

Marjorie Kruvand, PhD, is an associate professor and director of the masters in science in Global Strategic Communication program at the School of Communication at Loyola University Chicago. Previously, she was a senior vice president and partner specializing in health and science communication at FleishmanHillard, one of the world's leading communication agencies; a science and environmental reporter at the *St. Louis Post-Dispatch*; and a Knight Science Journalism Fellow at MIT. She received her PhD from the Missouri School of Journalism at the University of Missouri. Her research focuses on health and science communication, including mass communication of bioethical issues and the dynamics between public relations professionals and journalists.

Lisa M. Lee, PhD, MA, MS, is the executive director of the Presidential Commission for the Study of Bioethical Issues. Lee, who has a PhD from Johns Hopkins University, an MA in educational psychology from the

University of Colorado-Denver, and an MS in bioethics from Alden March Bioethics Institute at Albany Medical College, is an epidemiologist and public health ethicist. The focus of Lee's current work is bioethics pedagogy and public health ethics. Her prior work at the U.S. Centers for Disease Control and Prevention (CDC) included the ethics of public health surveillance, privacy and public health data use, and infectious disease epidemiology. During her 14-year career at CDC, she held several leadership positions, including serving as the agency's assistant science officer and director of the Office of Scientific Integrity. Lee is the lead editor of *Principles and Practice of Public Health Surveillance*, 3rd ed. (Oxford University Press, 2010). She has authored numerous publications in both science and ethics and serves as associate editor for the *Journal of Bioethical Inquiry* and *Public Health Reviews*. Dr. Lee serves on the Executive Board of Association for Practical and Professional Ethics and is an adjunct professor at the Center for Biomedical Ethics Education and Research at Albany Medical College, where she teaches ethics. She is the recipient of the 2014 Pellegrino Medal for excellence in bioethics.

Maimuna (Maia) S. Majumder is an engineering systems PhD student at MIT and computational epidemiology research fellow at HealthMap. Before coming to MIT, she earned a bachelor of science in engineering science and a masters of public health in epidemiology and biostatistics at Tufts University. Her research interests involve probabilistic modeling, Bayesian statistics, and "systems epidemiology" in the context of emerging infectious diseases. She also enjoys exploring novel techniques for data procurement, writing about data for the general public, and creating meaningful data visualizations. She's on Twitter at @maiamajumder.

Alexandra L. Phelan (Twitter: @alexandraphelan) is an adjunct professor in law, doctor of juridical science candidate, and Sir John Monash Scholar at Georgetown University Law Center in Washington, DC. Ms. Phelan's doctoral research examines the global law and governance of infectious diseases, including issues of international law, human rights, and global health security. Ms. Phelan holds a master of laws (with merit) from the Australian National University (Canberra, Australia) specializing in international law, and a bachelor of biomedical science/bachelor of laws (with honors) double degree from Monash University (Melbourne, Australia), specializing in international law and health human rights in her legal studies and infectious diseases in her biomedical science studies. Ms. Phelan previously worked as a solicitor at the global law firm King & Wood Mallesons, and has consulted for the World Health Organization and in the legal division at Gavi, the Vaccine Alliance. She is an associate fellow of the Royal Commonwealth Society, 2015 Emerging Leader in Biosecurity Initiative Fellow, Next-Generation Global Health Security Leader, and previously served as a director on Monash University's board of directors, University Council.

Annette Rid is a senior lecturer in Bioethics and Society at the Department of Social Science, Health, and Medicine at King's College London. Trained in medicine, philosophy, and bioethics in Germany, Switzerland, and the US, Annette's research interests span issues in research ethics, clinical ethics, and justice in health and health care. Annette has published widely in medical journals (e.g., *Lancet, JAMA*) and bioethics journals (e.g., *Journal of Medical Ethics, Hastings Center Report*). She has served as an advisor, among others, for the World Health Organization, the World Medical Association, and the Council of International Organizations of Medical Sciences. At King's, Annette has led the new master's degree program in bioethics and society as one of its inaugural co-directors. For more information, please see www.kcl.ac.uk/sshm and follow @anetrid on Twitter.

Cristine Russell is an award-winning journalist and educator who has written about science, public health, medicine, and the environment for more than three decades. She is a senior fellow at Harvard Kennedy School's Belfer Center for Science and International Affairs and an adjunct lecturer in public policy focusing on the media, climate, and energy. Russell, a former *Washington Post* national science and health reporter, is a freelance science writer, *Columbia Journalism Review* contributing editor, and contributor to publications such as *Scientific American* and the *Atlantic* online. Her work often addresses controversial issues at the intersection of science and public policy. Russell is a past president of two major American science-writing organizations: the National Association of Science Writers and the Council for the Advancement of Science Writing, and is co-chair of the Organizing Committee for the 2017 World Conference of Science Journalists in San Francisco. She has led efforts to improve media coverage and communication about global science to the general public and has also worked to promote leadership opportunities for women in science and journalism. Russell is a fellow of the American Association for the Advancement of Science and chair of the AAAS Section on General Interest in Science and Engineering. She is on the Commonwealth Fund board and has served on numerous other boards in journalism and education. Russell is a Phi Beta Kappa graduate in biology from Mills College. She can be found on Twitter at @russellcris.

Lara Schwarz studied Environment concentrating in Ecological Determinants of Health at McGill University. Her research interests include the social and environmental influences of infectious diseases. She first starting working on Ebola virus disease during the 2014 West Africa epidemic when she collaborated with Dr Bausch to write about it while he was working on the ground in Guinea. Lara now works as a Technical Officer in The Department of Pandemic and Epidemic Diseases at the World Health Organization, and continues to be involved with projects concerning Ebola and other zoonotic viruses.

Laura Seay is assistant professor of government at Colby College. Her research centers on questions at the intersection of conflict and development and the provision of public goods by non-state actors in Africa's fragile states. Her recent and current projects include a study of non-state actors and state reconstruction programs in the Democratic Republic of Congo, an evaluation of a World Bank-financed pilot program designed to improve use of clinical health care and maternal and child mortality rates in Nigeria, and a book project on the effects of American advocacy movements on U.S. policy in six African states. Seay serves on the executive board of the African Politics Conference Group and is co-contributing editor for Africa content at The Monkey Cage, a blog on politics and political science at the *Washington Post* (https://www.washingtonpost.com/news/monkey-cage/). Her work has been published in the *Review of African Political Economy*, *Perspectives on Politics*, and several edited volumes.

Michael J. Selgelid is director of Monash University's Centre for Human Bioethics and the World Health Organization (WHO) Collaborating Centre for Bioethics therein, and an adjunct professor in the School of Public Health and Preventative Medicine. He additionally holds an appointment as Monash-Warwick Honorary Professor in the Department of Politics and International Studies at the University of Warwick (UK). His main research focus is public health ethics, with emphasis on ethical issues associated with biotechnology and infectious disease. He has well over 100 publications in bioethics. He co-authored *Ethical and Philosophical Consideration of the Dual-Use Dilemma in the Biological Sciences* (Springer, 2008) and co-edited *On The Dual Uses of Science and Ethics: Principles, Practices, and Prospects* (ANU Press, 2013); *Ethics and Security Aspects of Infectious Disease Control: Interdisciplinary Perspectives* (Ashgate, 2012); *Emergency Ethics* (Ashgate, 2012); *Infectious Disease Ethics* (Springer, 2011); *Health Rights* (Ashgate, 2010); and *Ethics and Infectious Disease* (Blackwell, 2006). Michael earned a BS in biomedical engineering from Duke University and a PhD in philosophy from the University of California, San Diego, under the supervision of Philip Kitcher.

Tara C. Smith is an associate professor of epidemiology at Kent State University in Ohio. Dr. Smith's research focuses on zoonotic infections (infections that are transferred between animals and humans, such as Ebola). Her work has been profiled in many major publications, including *Science, Nature,* and *The New York Times*. Dr. Smith is also very active in science communication and outreach. She has maintained a science blog for 10 years and has written books on group A streptococcus, group B streptococcus, and Ebola. She also writes about infectious disease for Slate, Mic, and other sites. Find her on Twitter at @aetiology.

Armand Sprecher is an emergency physician and epidemiologist who has worked with Médecins Sans Frontières since 1997. He has been involved with filovirus outbreak response since 2000, including working in the field during the outbreaks in Uganda in 2000, Angola in 2005, the Democratic Republic of the Congo in 2007, and the outbreak in West Africa. Between outbreaks, aside from filovirus disease issues, Armand works mostly on health informatics. Armand has also worked with the International Medical Corps and the CDC's Epidemic Intelligence Service.

Index

Basic Bioethics

Arthur Caplan, editor

Books Acquired under the Editorship of Glenn McGee and Arthur Caplan

Peter A. Ubel, *Pricing Life: Why It's Time for Health Care Rationing*

Mark G. Kuczewski and Ronald Polansky, eds., *Bioethics: Ancient Themes in Contemporary Issues*

Suzanne Holland, Karen Lebacqz, and Laurie Zoloth, eds., *The Human Embryonic Stem Cell Debate: Science, Ethics, and Public Policy*

Gita Sen, Asha George, and Piroska Östlin, eds., *Engendering International Health: The Challenge of Equity*

Carolyn McLeod, *Self-Trust and Reproductive Autonomy*

Lenny Moss, *What Genes Can't Do*

Jonathan D. Moreno, ed., *In the Wake of Terror: Medicine and Morality in a Time of Crisis*

Glenn McGee, ed., *Pragmatic Bioethics, 2d edition*

Timothy F. Murphy, *Case Studies in Biomedical Research Ethics*

Mark A. Rothstein, ed., *Genetics and Life Insurance: Medical Underwriting and Social Policy*

Kenneth A. Richman, *Ethics and the Metaphysics of Medicine: Reflections on Health and Beneficence*

David Lazer, ed., *DNA and the Criminal Justice System: The Technology of Justice*

Harold W. Baillie and Timothy K. Casey, eds., *Is Human Nature Obsolete? Genetics, Bioengineering, and the Future of the Human Condition*

Robert H. Blank and Janna C. Merrick, eds., *End-of-Life Decision Making: A Cross-National Study*

Norman L. Cantor, *Making Medical Decisions for the Profoundly Mentally Disabled*

Margrit Shildrick and Roxanne Mykitiuk, eds., *Ethics of the Body: Post-Conventional Challenges*

Alfred I. Tauber, *Patient Autonomy and the Ethics of Responsibility*

David H. Brendel, *Healing Psychiatry: Bridging the Science/Humanism Divide*

Jonathan Baron, *Against Bioethics*

Michael L. Gross, *Bioethics and Armed Conflict: Moral Dilemmas of Medicine and War*

Karen F. Greif and Jon F. Merz, *Current Controversies in the Biological Sciences: Case Studies of Policy Challenges from New Technologies*

Deborah Blizzard, *Looking Within: A Sociocultural Examination of Fetoscopy*

Ronald Cole-Turner, ed., *Design and Destiny: Jewish and Christian Perspectives on Human Germline Modification*

Holly Fernandez Lynch, *Conflicts of Conscience in Health Care: An Institutional Compromise*

Mark A. Bedau and Emily C. Parke, eds., *The Ethics of Protocells: Moral and Social Implications of Creating Life in the Laboratory*

Jonathan D. Moreno and Sam Berger, eds., *Progress in Bioethics: Science, Policy, and Politics*

Eric Racine, *Pragmatic Neuroethics: Improving Understanding and Treatment of the Mind-Brain*

Martha J. Farah, ed., *Neuroethics: An Introduction with Readings*

Jeremy R. Garrett, ed., *The Ethics of Animal Research: Exploring the Controversy*

Books Acquired under the Editorship of Arthur Caplan

Sheila Jasanoff, ed., *Reframing Rights: Bioconstitutionalism in the Genetic Age*

Christine Overall, *Why Have Children? The Ethical Debate*

Yechiel Michael Barilan, *Human Dignity, Human Rights, and Responsibility: The New Language of Global Bioethics and Bio-Law*

Tom Koch, *Thieves of Virtue: When Bioethics Stole Medicine*

Timothy F. Murphy, *Ethics, Sexual Orientation, and Choices about Children*

Daniel Callahan, *In Search of the Good: A Life in Bioethics*

Robert Blank, *Intervention in the Brain: Politics, Policy, and Ethics*

Gregory E. Kaebnick and Thomas H. Murray, eds., *Synthetic Biology and Morality: Artificial Life and the Bounds of Nature*

Dominic A. Sisti, Arthur L. Caplan, and Hila Rimon-Greenspan, eds., *Applied Ethics in Mental Healthcare: An Interdisciplinary Reader*

Barbara K. Redman, *Research Misconduct Policy in Biomedicine: Beyond the Bad-Apple Approach*

Russell Blackford, *Humanity Enhanced: Genetic Choice and the Challenge for Liberal Democracies*

Nicholas Agar, *Truly Human Enhancement: A Philosophical Defense of Limits*

Bruno Perreau, *The Politics of Adoption: Gender and the Making of French Citizenship*

Carl Schneider, *The Censor's Hand: The Misregulation of Human-Subject Research*

Lydia S. Dugdale, ed., *Dying in the Twenty-First Century: Towards a New Ethical Framework for the Art of Dying Well*

John D. Lantos and Diane S. Lauderdale, *Preterm Babies, Fetal Patients, and Childbearing Choices*

Harris Wiseman, *The Myth of the Moral Brain: The Limits of Moral Enhancement*

Nicholas G. Evans, Tara C. Smith, and Maimuna S. Majumder, eds., *Ebola's Message: Public Health and Medicine in the Twenty-First Century*